THE SABBATH.

BY

CHARLES ELLIOTT,

PROFESSOR OF BIBLICAL LITERATURE AND EXEGESIS IN THE PRESBYTERIAN THEOLOGICAL SEMINARY OF THE NORTH-WEST, CHICAGO, ILL.

PHILADELPHIA:
PRESBYTERIAN BOARD OF PUBLICATION,
No. 821 CHESTNUT STREET.

WESTCOTT & THOMSON,
STEREOTYPERS, PHILADA.

PREFACE.

THE only apology for the publication of this little volume is the importance of the subject that it discusses. The Sabbath is an institution intimately connected with the highest interests of religion, and consequently with all that is most precious to humanity. It also contributes to man's physical comfort and secular prosperity. Every attempt, therefore, to weaken its obligation should be resisted; and every false view promulgated respecting it should be refuted. If this little treatise shall, in any way, contribute to that end, to Him be the praise, whose voice proclaimed from the top of Sinai: "Remember the Sabbath day, to keep it holy."

THE AUTHOR.

CONTENTS.

PAGE
PREFACE.. 3

PART I.

THE LAW OF THE SABBATH HAS ITS FOUNDATION IN OUR NATURE.

CHAPTER I.

SECTION I.

Meaning of the term—The Law of the Sabbath founded in our constitution, physical, intellectual, and moral.. 9

SECTION II.

The Physical or Physiological Advantages of the Sabbath........................ 13

SECTION III.

The Intellectual Advantages of the Sabbath.. 19

SECTION IV.

The Moral and Spiritual Advantages of the Sabbath........................ 23

CHAPTER II.

THE SOCIAL ADVANTAGES OF THE SABBATH.

SECTION I.

The Family.. 27

SECTION II.

PAGE

The Community 34

SECTION III.

Summary of the preceding sections 38

PART II.

SECTION I.

Institution of the Sabbath 41

SECTION II.

The Sabbath a Moral Institution 49

SECTION III.

Change of the Sabbath from the Seventh day of the week to the First 59

SECTION IV.

The Perpetuity of the Sabbath 66

SECTION V.

Summary 74

PART III.

THE SANCTIFICATION OF THE SABBATH.

SECTION I.

Preliminary Observations 76

SECTION II.

The Sabbath is to be kept in such a way as to perpetuate the Knowledge and Worship of Jehovah 79

SECTION III.

PAGE

The Sabbath is to be Sanctified by attending to the Private Exercises of Religion.......... 85

SECTION IV.

The Sabbath is to be Sanctified by Bodily Rest, and by intermitting such Intellectual Employments as are not immediately connected with the services of Religion.......... 90

SECTION V.

The Duty of the state with reference to the Sanctification of the Sabbath. 94

SECTION VI.

Concluding Remarks.......... 106

THE SABBATH.

PART I.

THE LAW OF THE SABBATH HAS ITS FOUNDATION IN OUR NATURE.

CHAPTER I.

SECTION I.

MEANING OF THE TERM—THE LAW OF THE SABBATH FOUNDED IN OUR CONSTITUTION, PHYSICAL, INTELLECTUAL, AND MORAL.

THE word Sabbath is of Hebrew origin, and signifies rest. It is not synonymous with Sunday. The former designates that day of the seven, which is set apart for rest and worship; the latter is the name of the first day of the week. This distinction is observed in the Homilies of the established Church of England. "So, if we will be the children of our heavenly Father, we must be careful to keep the Christian Sabbath day, which is the Sunday." The distinction seems to be that the term Sabbath is applied to the institution of sacred rest, and that Sunday is the name of the day. Notwithstanding this distinction, they are often used synonymously, both in the United States and in England. It is better, however, to retain the use of Sabbath, or to employ the designation, Lord's Day, as it suggests the idea of holy time.

Our Lord said to the Pharisees when they asked him why his disciples did that which was not lawful on the Sabbath day, by plucking the ears of corn in the fields through which they were passing: "The Sabbath was made for man, and not man for the Sabbath."

These words teach that the Sabbath was designed for man's advantage, and imply that its proper observance is not detrimental to his best interests, but highly productive of them; and this being the case they further imply that there is an adaptation of the Sabbatical institution to man's nature. "The Sabbath was made for man." It was designed to meet his physical, intellectual, and spiritual wants. Its law is founded in his constitution. This we will readily perceive if we consider the wants which the institution of the Sabbath meets. All men need rest for their bodies, and it would be a difficult matter to prove that a seventh portion of our time is too much. Now, were there no day set apart for cessation from labour, many would be deprived of that periodical relaxation from their regular routine of duty, the uninterrupted continuance of which exhausts the bodily powers, and thus impairs health. The same thing might be affirmed of those lower animals that are used as beasts of draught and burden, for they require rest as well as man.

Analogies to this law obtain throughout inanimate nature. There are seasons of rest for the soil and for trees. Winter locks the earth in its embrace, but its frosts and snows prepare fresh nutriment for the flowers of spring. The soil is thus preserved from exhaustion by a period of annual repose.

Man is an intellectual being, and needs knowledge, especially, knowledge of God, of himself, and of his relations to God. To acquire this knowledge some portion of time is necessary; but without a Sabbath many would be deprived of the opportunity of acquiring it, and consequently would remain in ignorance of their highest duty. By affording this opportunity to every one, the Sabbath meets man's highest intellectual wants, and thus shows its adaptation to his intellectual nature.

Man is also possessed of conscience and will, and is influenced by motives. He is an immortal being, placed in this world to prepare for a higher and better state of existence. To apply spiritual truths to his conscience and make them motives to influence his will, he must have time to withdraw his mind from secular employments, and fix it upon these truths, and to place himself under the influence of things that are unseen and eternal. Nothing is so favourable to this as the quiet of a well-spent Sabbath, when the serenity, peace, and solemnity of the heavenly world seem to invest all things around us. The very air seems to breathe of heaven. The eye seems to pierce deeper into the blue expanse above us. The sun seems clothed in fresh glory, and when the stars of evening rise, they seem to shine with additional lustre. This may be all imagination. It doubtless is; but it is the imagination of one who has been conversing with God. It is not the air, the heavens, the sun, and the stars that are changed; but the change is in the mind, and it sees all things beautiful. A day that affords an opportunity for those elevated contemplations which produce such a change in the mind, must be admirably adapted to the culture of man's spiritual nature.

We may conclude, from these observations, that the law of the Sabbath has its foundation in man's physical, intellectual, and moral constitution, and consequently that its proper observance is productive of his highest benefit. When we keep the Sabbath as it ought to be kept, we are merely acting in obedience to a law, the final end of which is to promote our physical, intellectual, and moral well-being; and the violation of which is a violation of that well-being.

We have merely indicated in what way the Sabbath promotes our welfare, by showing that its law is laid in our constitution. It may be well to enter into detail on this point, and fortify ourselves by facts. These facts are abundant, and drawn from a great variety of sources.

We will first consider its advantages to man as a day of rest, for the purpose of invigorating the body, preserving it in health, and prolonging life; or, in other words, its physiological advantages. On this point we have the concurrent testimony of the highest authorities.

SECTION II.

THE PHYSICAL, OR PHYSIOLOGICAL ADVANTAGES OF THE SABBATH.

On this point the writer will make a free use of some facts contained in the first number of the *Sabbath Manual.*

In the year 1832 the British House of Commons appointed a committee to investigate the effects of labouring seven days in a week compared with those of labouring six, and resting one. This committee, composed of statesmen of the greatest eminence, such as Sir Robert Peel, Lord Morpeth, Sir Robert Inglis, Sir Andrew Agnew, and Sir Thomas Baring, with many others,—examined a great number of witnesses of various professions and employments. Among these witnesses was an acute and experienced physician, Dr. Farre of London. Dr. F., previous to the time of giving his testimony, had practised medicine between thirty and forty years; and during the early part of his life, as the physician of a public medical institution, had had charge of one of the most populous districts of London. He had had occasion to observe the effects of the observance and non-observance of the seventh as a day of rest during this time. He had considered its uses from a medical point of view, and observed its abuses as manifested in labour and dissipation; and his testimony, as a physician, was, that medically viewed, the Sabbath is a most beneficent institution.

"As a day of rest," said Dr. Farre, "I view it as a day of *compensation* for the inadequate restorative power of the body under *continued* labour and excitement. A physician always has respect to the restorative power; because if once this be lost, his healing office is at end. A physician is anxious to preserve the balance of circulation, as necessary to the restorative power of the body. The ordinary exertions of man *run down* the circulation every day of his life; and the first general law of his nature, by which God prevents man from destroying himself, is the alternating of day and night, that repose may succeed action. But, although the night apparently equalizes the circulation, yet it does not sufficiently restore its balance for the attainment of a long life. Hence, *one day in seven*, by the bounty of Providence, is thrown in as a day of *compensation*, to perfect by its repose the animal system. You may easily," continued the Doctor, "determine this question, as a matter of fact, by trying it on beasts of burden. Take that fine animal, the horse, and work him to the full extent of his powers every day in the week, or give him rest one day in seven, and you will soon perceive, by the superior vigour with which he performs his functions on the other six days, that his rest is necessary to his well-being. Man possesses a superior nature, is borne along by the very vigour of his mind; so that the injury of *continued* diurnal exertion and excitement on the animal system is not so immediately apparent as it is in the brute; but in the long run he breaks down more suddenly; it abridges the length of his life; and that vigour of his old age, which (as to mere animal power) ought to be the object of his preservation." The same witness says that "researches in physiology, by the analogy of the working of Providence in nature, will show that the Divine commandment is not to be considered an arbitrary enactment, but as an appointment necessary to man."

The celebrated Wilberforce ascribed the continuance of his life, for so long a time, under such a pressure of cares and labours, in no small degree, to his conscientious and habitual observance of the Sabbath. He considered it a blessed day, which "allows us a precious interval wherein to pause, to come out from the thickets of worldly concerns, and give ourselves up to heavenly and spiritual objects. Observation and my own experience," said Mr. W., "have convinced me that there is a special blessing on a right employment of these intervals."

During the life of this celebrated Christian and statesman, Sir Samuel Romilly, Solicitor General of England, and Lord Castlereagh, terminated their lives each by his own hand. The impression on Mr. W's. mind was that it was the effect of continued wear of mind occasioned by the non-observance of the Sabbath on the part of these two celebrated men. When endeavours were made to prevail upon the lawyers of London to give up Sabbath consultation, Sir S. Romilly would not concur; and Lord Castlereagh was so engrossed with politics that he allowed his mind no relaxation. The constant recurring of the same reflections dethroned his reason, and led to the commission of the fatal act, which deprived him of his life. "He was the last man in the world," remarked Mr. Wilberforce, "who appeared likely to be carried away into the commission of such an act; so cool, so self-possessed."

In the same testimony concur such men as Thomas Sewall, M. D., Professor of Pathology and the Practice of Medicine in the Columbian College, Washington, D. C.; Dr. Mussey, Professor of Surgery in the Ohio Medical College; Dr. Harrison of the same institution; Dr. Alden, of Massachusetts; and the New Haven Medical Association, composed of twenty-five physicians, among whom were the professors of the medical college.

The first of these remarks: "While I consider it the more important design of the institution of the Sabbath, to assist in religious devotion and advance man's spiritual welfare, I have long held the opinion that one of its chief benefits has reference to his *physical and intellectual* constitution; affording him, as it does, one day in seven for the renovation of his exhausted energies of body and mind; a proportion of time small enough, according to the results of my observation, for the accomplishment of this object."

Dr. Mussey remarks: "The Sabbath should be regarded as a most *benevolent* institution, adapted alike to the physical, mental, and moral wants of man. The experiment has been made with animals, and the value of one day's work in seven, for those that labour, in recruiting their energies and prolonging their activity, has been established beyond a doubt. In addition to constant bodily labour, the corroding influence of incessant *mental* exertion and solicitude cannot fail to induce *premature* decay, and to shorten life. And there cannot be a reasonable doubt, that under the due observance of the Sabbath, life would, on the average, be prolonged more than one-seventh of its whole period; that is, more than seven years in fifty."

The other eminent physicians, and the New Haven Medical Association, express the same sentiments.

To these testimonies might be added those of men of all professions and employments—merchants, tradesmen, fishermen, men employed on steamboats and public works,—who all concur in the same thing.

These testimonies are not unsupported by facts. Interesting experiments have been made upon both men and animals to test the salutary nature of the law of the Sabbath, and they have always resulted in the conclusion that both require the rest of the sacred day.

One of these experiments was made in a large flouring establishment. For a number of years the mills were worked seven days a week. The superintendent was then changed. He ordered the men to stop the works at eleven o'clock on Saturday night, and not to start them till one o'clock on Monday morning, thus allowing a full Sabbath every week. And the same men, during the year, actually ground fifty thousand bushels more than had ever been ground, in a single year, in that establishment before. The men having been permitted to cleanse themselves, put on their best apparel, rest from worldly business, go with their families to the house of God, and devote the Sabbath to its appropriate duties,—were more healthy, punctual, moral, and diligent. They lost less time in drinking, dissipation and quarrels. They were more clear-headed and whole-hearted; knew better how to do things, and were more disposed to do them in the right way.

Another experiment was tried on a hundred and twenty horses. They were employed for years, seven days in the week. But they became unhealthy, and finally died so fast that the owner thought it too expensive, and put them on a six days' arrangement. After this he was not obliged to replenish them one-fourth part as often as before. Instead of sinking continually, his horses came up again, and lived longer than they could have done on the other plan.

A manufacturing company, which had been accustomed to carry their goods to market with their own teams, kept them employed seven days in a week, as that was the time in which they could go to the market and return. But by permitting the teams to rest on the Sabbath, they found that they could drive them the same distance in six days, that they had formerly done in seven, and with the same keeping preserve them in better order.

These testimonies and facts fully show the salutary influence of the Sabbath upon the physical constitutions of both man and the lower animals. As a day of rest it is "a day of *compensation* for the inadequate restorative power of the body under *continued* labour and excitement."

SECTION III.

THE INTELLECTUAL ADVANTAGES OF THE SABBATH.

The mind requires repose as well as the body, and this repose a well-spent Sabbath affords. It is not necessary, in this connection, to discuss the question whether the mind itself becomes fatigued, or whether it is merely the bodily organs, through which it operates, that become exhausted by labour, and are invigorated by rest. Nor is it necessary for the rest of the mind that it sink into a state of inactivity, in which all its faculties become dormant, or listless. The highest refreshment to the mind is oftentimes furnished by directing it to something new, something that will relieve it from its usual routine of thought, and afford it an opportunity for the exercise of the imagination and the emotions. When worn out by labour, the sight of a beautiful landscape, or of a lake embosomed among hills, or of some work of art, will rouse it from its languor and fatigue, and fill it with buoyant feelings and exhilarating delight.

The opportunity of directing the mind to something new is furnished by nothing so well as by the institution of the Sabbath. It interrupts the ordinary pursuits of man, and turns his mind to the contemplation of the most glorious and soul-inspiring truths within the whole range of thought. God, heaven, eternity, the soul and its immortal destinies, all that is beautiful and holy on earth, are thoughts strictly in unison with the sacred character of the day, and in fact suggested by its very institution and end. On it God rested. It is to us a type of the heavenly rest, which remains for the people of God. And when, on this sacred day, we rise above the earth and see the visions of the Almighty, what inspiration do we feel; what fresh vigour in the divine life, what grandeur of thought, what intensity of purpose do we acquire. And if any are mourners amidst the decay of all things earthly, what comfort does it inspire to have such a blessed opportunity to look beyond this world of change to that land

> ——"of pure delight,
> Where saints immortal reign,
> Where endless day excludes the night,
> And pleasures banish pain."

Then such may feel, even here, the breath of its everlasting spring, and inhale the odour of its never withering flowers.

It is true these holy and elevating influences are not confined to the Sabbath; but may be enjoyed by the Christian on other days, for God is always near to those that call upon him; and the consolations of his grace are vouchsafed, at all seasons, to such as seek him with a contrite heart. Yet it cannot be denied that there is something in the holy quiet of the Sabbath, something in its associations, something in the very fact of its institution, which renders it eminently fitted to inspire and cherish the holiest thoughts, and to make it a source of the richest intellectual and spiritual blessings.

Now this is just such a rest as the mind needs, a rest from weariness and care, a rest from worldly occupations and pursuits, a rest from meditation upon things visible and temporal, in the calm and elevated contemplation upon the unseen and eternal.

Meditation upon these lofty truths cannot fail to cultivate man's intellectual as well as his spiritual nature; and hence a Sabbath-keeping people are always intelligent. Men, who in the course of three-score years and ten, spend ten years, as they may do, if they spend their Sabbaths as they ought, in studying the sublimest truths that can occupy the mind, if possessed of ordinary capacity, must acquire a large amount of knowledge eminently serviceable to them in every walk of life; for the truths of religion are not mere speculations, but practical principles to direct us in all the duties arising out of our various relations.

Add to the meditation upon these truths the reading of the Bible, of good books, and the listening to public instruction from men of learning and intelligence, and it will be at once seen, that the influence of the Sabbath—when devoted to its legitimate ends—upon intellectual culture cannot be overrated. It affords an opportunity for the acquisition of that knowledge, without which the will is deprived of its strongest motives, and law of its highest sanctions.

This part of the subject is susceptible of ample illustration by examples. Let it suffice to refer to the superior mental vigour and proficiency of those young men at college, who exchange their ordinary studies for the proper duties of the Sabbath, compared with those who pursue their studies on that sacred day. Professors in colleges have doubtless observed the fact.

SECTION IV.

THE MORAL AND SPIRITUAL ADVANTAGES OF THE SABBATH.

These have been alluded to in the preceding section; but they are sufficiently important to require a separate discussion. Indeed, they are the most important advantages secured by the day of holy rest.

Moral, contradistinguished from *spiritual*, relates to duty or obligation. It pertains to those motives and actions of which right and wrong, virtue and vice, may be affirmed or denied. It relates to the practice, manners, or conduct of men, so far as those are the subjects of law. *Spiritual*, as distinguished from *moral*, pertains to the soul and its affections, as influenced by the Holy Spirit. It includes the moral; but the moral does not necessarily include the spiritual.

The moral advantages of the Sabbath commend themselves to the most superficial thinker. The very observance of a day, out of respect to our own well-being, is itself a great moral benefit, as it habituates the mind to thoughts of self-preservation and bodily comfort. Add to this the observance of it out of regard to the authority of God, and the moral advantage is heightened, because the mind is brought under the influence of the unseen and eternal. While under this influence, and freed from worldly avocations, it is prepared and has opportunity, to consider questions of duty, to weigh motives, to determine the quality of actions, and to form plans and resolutions of doing good. No other day, on account of the various and necessary occupations of life, can be so favourable for these things as the holy Sabbath.

Its spiritual advantages are chiefly, though not entirely, confined to the Christian. The impenitent are often led, by its institution, by its sacred associations and holy duties, to think of "that rest which remaineth to the people of God," to feel their need of preparation for it, and to apply for salvation to Him, who "taketh away the sin of the world." The Sabbath is a constant memorial of the heavenly rest, and a standing invitation to all that are weary and heavy laden to seek it; and many have accepted the invitation, and found the rest for which they sighed.

To the Christian it is a foretaste of heaven. During its sacred hours, he can draw off his mind from those worldly thoughts and distracting cares which grow out of his pursuits on other days, and hold communion with the Father of his spirit. He can meditate, without interruption, on the riches of the inheritance of the saints in glory, on the love of God, on the grace and condescension of Christ, and on the consolation of the Holy Spirit. While thus occupied, his soul is often wafted upward on the wings of faith and hope, until he imagines himself mingling with the blissful throng in the presence of the ineffable glory. And when the glorious vision passes, and he feels himself still an inhabitant of the earth, how often does he breathe out his soul, in the language of the poet:

"Who, who would live alway, away from his God;
Away from yon heaven, that blissful abode,
Where the rivers of pleasure flow o'er the bright plains,
And the noontide of glory eternally reigns:

"Where the saints of all ages in harmony meet,
Their Saviour and brethren transported to greet;
While the anthems of rapture unceasingly roll,
And the smile of the Lord is the feast of the soul?"

But the exercises of the Christian are not always of a rapturous kind, even on the Sabbath. The child of God often has his doubts and fears, his troubles and sorrows. When thus affected, what a blessed privilege it is for him to have the opportunity of self-examination, of communion with God in the closet, of confessing his sins and supplicating the Divine forgiveness, of reading the Bible, and pondering its precious promises, of going to the house of God and listening to the preaching of the word, of conferring with other Christians, and learning that his trials are not peculiar. If he has been faithful in these things, peace has returned to his mind, and he has been enabled to say, with the Psalmist: "Why art thou cast down, O my soul? and why art thou disquieted within me? hope in God: for I shall yet praise him, who is the health of my countenance, and my God."

The writer does not intend to convey the idea that these holy exercises and sacred privileges are confined to the Sabbath; but he does intend to convey the idea that there is something in the very institution and associations of the Sabbath favourable to them, and in fact suggestive of them. Were there no Sabbath, some of them could not be enjoyed at all, and others would be in danger of being neglected. If, with the inestimable privilege of one day in seven for such holy and elevating exercises, Christians are so feeble in the divine life, what would they be without it? God only can tell.

We must conclude, then, that the Sabbath is the source of incalculable moral and spiritual advantages, that without it morality and religion would scarcely exist.

CHAPTER II.

THE SOCIAL ADVANTAGES OF THE SABBATH.

SECTION I.

THE FAMILY.

THE Sabbath is a beneficent family institution. Without it the great end of the family could not be accomplished. What is that end? The mere increase of the human species? That might multiply only wickedness and woe. It is to raise up a "godly seed." "And did not he make one? Yet had he the residue of the Spirit. And wherefore one? That he might seek a godly seed. Therefore take heed to your spirit, and let none deal treacherously against the wife of his youth." (Malachi ii. 15.) In a state of innocence, amidst the delights of Paradise, God instituted marriage and the Sabbath, the former to perpetuate the race, the latter to preserve it in its highest state of earthly blessedness.

How does the Sabbath minister to this end? To answer this question, it will be necessary to consider the reciprocal duties of parents and children, so that the connection between these duties and the Sabbatical institution may be more clearly comprehended.

The duties that the parent owes to the child are

maintenance, government, and education. The first has no direct or necessary connection with the point under discussion, and may, therefore, be dismissed. The other two depend, for their faithful and fullest discharge, very much upon the proper observance of the Sabbath.

"The family is a little society, a miniature state; and every society, every state, must have its laws, its government." It is the duty of the divinely constituted head, the father, or, in case of his absence or death, the mother, to administer that government, and to enforce these laws. The very first law of the family is obedience to parental authority in the Lord; to honour father and mother. Submission to this law is obligatory on the child, and must be required by the parent. If insubordination is allowed on the part of the parents, the consequences to the child may prove fatal to its interests, both temporal and eternal. Hence it is a duty which the parent owes to the state and to God, to teach his child respect for rightful authority and submission to it. It is in this way that children are trained for useful service in the world, that the family becomes "a nursery for higher and broader spheres of action. In it the seeds are planted, and the germs are nurtured, which are to have their full development, and bear their fruit in future years, and in other worlds." This is the end to be aimed at in family government; and it is an end which, as a general rule, will be accomplished, if that government is properly enforced. But if there is any laxity, or unfaithfulness on the part of the parent, in this respect, the child goes forth from his father's house, unfitted to assume those solemn responsibilities which will devolve upon him as a member of society, or as the head of a family, should he ever become one.

The duty of a parent is not limited to the government of his children: he must also educate them. This education must have reference to their training, physical, intellectual, and moral. The importance of possessing a good physical constitution is universally acknowledged; this the parent should endeavour to secure for the child by the use of such means as will best develop the bodily powers. Simultaneously with this, the intellect must be trained to habits of thought and reflection; useful knowledge must be imparted, so that the mind may receive its proper aliment, and all its faculties find their appropriate exercise.

But the most important branch of education is the moral. The heart of the child must be educated. On this depends his eternal happiness. He must be taught his relations to God and to his fellow-men and the duties arising out of these relations; and these duties must be enforced by the highest sanctions and by the most powerful motives. The parent is, moreover, responsible, in a great measure, for the religious faith of the child. It is too much the custom of the present day to allow children to grow up without any well-defined views of divine truth. There seems to be a fear, on the part of many parents, lest the minds of their children should become prejudiced, were they instructed in the doctrines of the Bible, especially as held by any one denomination of Christians. Hence they are left to form their own religious opinions, as inclination or circumstances may determine. Such neglect, on the part of the parent, is downright dishonesty, in case he holds any decided religious views. It is in effect saying that all beliefs are equally good. The Bible gives no countenance to such indifference. It enjoins upon parents to bring up their "children in the nurture and admonition of the Lord;" and upon children to "hear the instruction of a father and" to "attend to know understanding." (Ephes. vi. 4; Prov. iv. 1, 2.) And the Lord assigned as a reason, why he did not hide what he was about to do from Abraham, "For I know him, that he will command his children, and his household after him, and they shall keep the way of the Lord, to do justice and judgment."

These duties, on the part of the parent, imply reciprocal ones on the part of the child. If it is the duty of the parent to govern, it is the duty of the child to obey. If there is obligation resting on the parent to educate, the child must yield himself to be trained and guided. There are also duties arising out of the very relation of parent and child, which the latter is bound, by the highest considerations, to fulfil. To enumerate them is not necessary to the present purpose. They may be summed up in obedience, docility, and love.

The way is now open to see the intimate connection between family government and education, and the Sabbath institution.

It is an adage that example is more efficacious than precept. When the parent, therefore, in obedience to God's commandment, remembers the Sabbath day to keep it holy, he is using the very best means for securing wholesome family government. He thus most effectually impresses upon the mind of the child the ideas of law and obligation. He might enjoin precept upon precept, but unless his own example conformed to his teaching, the latter would be without effect. When the child sees the parent practically acknowledging the authority of God by keeping his commandments, it cannot fail to have awakened within it the feeling of reverence and a sense of duty. The idea of a moral government will be associated with its earliest recollections, with the dawn of reason, and will prove a salutary restraint during its whole future life.

The Sabbath moreover, by bringing together all the members of the family, under the eye and immediate control of the father, the fountain of household authority, affords a better opportunity for exercising domestic government, than any other portion of the week, when separation from one another much of the time interferes with the best plans of instruction and discipline, and secular affairs engross the attention. Occasional precept and example, without the presence of power to enforce them, might soon be forgotten. Hence the importance that the pupil should be under the eye and immediate direction of the teacher. This privilege in the case of the family the Sabbath secures.

If the Sabbath, when properly observed, tends to sustain domestic government, it no less tends to promote domestic education.

Let us view it in connection with the physical education of children. It affords them a day of rest from manual labour, or from school; an opportunity of cleansing themselves and putting on their best apparel; of attending Sabbath-school and church. All these things have a tendency to produce cheerfulness and equanimity of mind, to promote order and health. The effect can be no other than salutary to have a respite from their childish cares and sorrows, from their weekly tasks and toils, as they may have if their parents exact from them a proper observance of the Lord's day. These hours of holy time they will regard as the most pleasant of their lives, and they will learn to hail their return with delight.

To effect this the Sabbath must not be made to them, as it too often is by well-meaning but mistaken parents, a day of gloom, but a day of cheerfulness. They must be taught that it was designed to promote their physical comfort and well-being, and that they should use it in such a way as to accomplish that end.

But the Sabbath has higher aims than man's physical benefit. The culture of the soul is its chief design. How kind is God to give us a day for this purpose—a day without which many families would be deprived of the most ennobling influences that can be experienced in this world, and without which none would enjoy them in all their richness and power!

That the Lord's day is eminently fitted for this highest of all culture no candid man can doubt. The intellect is awakened by the associations and teachings of the day—teachings on subjects that require the most profound and patient thought—the power of conscience is increased by a constant sense of the obligations of divine law, the purest earthly affections are strengthened by the sweet and hallowed influences of the domestic hearth. In none but a Sabbath-keeping country could such a scene as that portrayed in the "Cotter's Saturday night" be laid. The father, mother, and children, some of whom are out at service, meet on the eve of the Sabbath, for the purpose of spending that holy day together as a family. After their frugal repast has been finished, and they have formed a circle round their cottage fire,

"The sire turns o'er wi' patriarchal grace,
The big ha' Bible, once his father's pride:
His bonnet rev'rently is laid aside,

His lyart haffets wearin' thin and bare;
Those strains that once did sweet in Zion glide,
He wales a portion with judicious care;
And, 'Let us worship God!' he says with solemn air.

"They chant their artless notes in simple guise;
They tune their hearts, by far the noblest aim;
Perhaps Dundee's wild warbling measures rise,
Or, plaintive Martyrs, worthy of the name;
Or noble Elgin beats the heavenward flame,
The sweetest far of Scotia's holy lays:
Compared with these, Italian trills are tame;
The tickled ears no heartfelt raptures raise;
Nae unison hae they with our Creator's praise."

After he has read a lesson from the sacred page,

"Then kneeling down, to heaven's Eternal King,
The *saint*, the *father*, and the *husband* prays:
Hope, 'springs exulting on triumphant wing,'
That *thus* they all shall meet in future days:
There, ever bask in uncreated rays,
No more to sigh, or shed the bitter tear,
Together hymning their Creator's praise,
In such society, yet still more dear;
While circling time moves round in an eternal sphere."

SECTION II.

THE COMMUNITY.

From the advantages of the Sabbath upon the individual and the family, it is easy and natural to pass to those upon the community. Communities are composed of individuals and families, consequently whatever benefits the latter must also benefit the former. The aggregate contains the sum of the several particulars; hence particular benefits make up the sum of the aggregate benefits.

The chief blessings of a community are intelligence, religion, morality, and good laws. The first three of these the institution of the Sabbath promotes directly, and indirectly secures the enactment of the last, with obedience to them.

It requires no wide induction of facts, no extended argument, to prove that the Sabbath, when properly observed, promotes intelligence. All the exercises, both public and private, peculiar to the day, tend to quicken the intellect and enlarge the views. The reading of the Bible and good books, the attendance upon public worship, and listening to discourses from able and learned men, and meditation upon the sublimest truths within the range of human thought, and that periodically, during the seventh portion of each man's lifetime, must, from the very nature of things, diffuse a degree of intelligence, which could never be attained, without the Sabbatical rest.

The connection between knowledge and religion is inseparable. Our Saviour said, "This is life eternal, that they might know thee, the only true God, and Jesus Christ, whom thou hast sent." Indeed, all true religion is based upon religious knowledge—a knowledge of the true God. To conserve and propagate this knowledge, the church has been organized, and ordinances of worship have been established. Her mission is to disciple all nations. In the fulfilment of this mission, God has been with her, and crowned her efforts with success. He has sent his Holy Spirit to render the preaching of his word effectual, to edify his people, to comfort their hearts, and to convert sinners. Much of the success of this high and holy work has been in connection with the observance of the Sabbath. Where there is no such observance, it is a rare thing to find vital godliness. Dead formality exists, and open, gross immorality pervades every grade of society. And this state of things is just in proportion to the extent of the desecration of the Sabbath.

If any are skeptical on this point, let them compare Roman Catholic countries with Protestant, and those Protestant countries where the Sabbath is generally and properly observed, with other Protestant countries, where it is not, and their skepticism will soon vanish.

True religion is the basis of sound morality; for morality consists in the performance of those duties that are enjoined by the divine law. But the fulfilment of this law is love, which is the very essence of religion. If religion, therefore, is lacking, the very ground element of all morality is wanting. The relation between religion and morality being so intimate, whatever promotes the interests of the one must promote the interests of the other. If the observance of the Sabbath, therefore, is essential to the prosperity of religion, it is no less so to that of morality.

This deduction is conformable to facts. Those communities in which the purest morality is found, are the religious, Sabbath-keeping communities. For proof of this, it is necessary only to refer to Scotland, the north of Ireland, England, and our own country. That the superior morality of these countries is the fruit of their evangelical religion, scarcely any one will have the hardihood to deny; that the vitality of their religion is preserved by keeping holy the Sabbath day will be almost as readily admitted, if the nature and object of the Sabbath are considered, together with the fact that its sanctification and true piety are seldom ever found separated.

It is not necessary to do more than merely to allude to the influence of all this upon legislation and good order. The laws of a country—especially of a free country—are a very good index of its moral theories and sentiments. If these are wrong, the laws will be of the same character, unless practical difficulties intervene to prevent the application of them in legislation. Hence the necessity of sound moral principles in order to secure the enactment of good laws. The practice of morality, consisting in cheerful and constant obedience to law, is no less necessary to good order. Such being the case, the connection between the sanctification of the Sabbath and the highest civil and political interests of a community is apparent.

What has been said in this section might be abundantly illustrated by an appeal to the facts of history, many of which will suggest themselves to the mind of the intelligent reader. To adduce them would cause the writer to transcend the limits which he has imposed upon himself. His chief aim is to state principles and illustrate them only far enough to draw attention to a much neglected, but very important, subject.

SECTION III.

SUMMARY OF THE PRECEDING SECTIONS.

In a field, whose limits are not visible, the labourer finds satisfaction in frequently looking behind him, to see how much of it he has brought under his cultivating hand. So it is with the student and writer. They experience both benefit and pleasure in reviewing the ground that they have passed over, and in determining clearly the precise point at which they have arrived. Let us take a brief review, that we may see more clearly the point that we have reached.

We have endeavoured to show that the law of the Sabbath is founded in the constitution of man, by the fact that it is necessary to his physical, intellectual, moral, and spiritual well-being. Its physical advantages are, that as a day of rest, it affords compensation for the inadequate restorative power of the body under continued labour and excitement; it gives repose, and promotes cleanliness and health.

To the intellect it affords an opportunity for agreeable change, for thought and reflection upon the loftiest truths that can occupy the mind, for availing itself of the instructions of able and learned men, and of good books; and for subjecting itself to all those quickening influences which the exercises of the Sabbath are fitted to produce.

It supplies man's spiritual need by affording him an opportunity of applying spiritual truths to his conscience, of making them motives to influence his will, and of placing himself more unreservedly than he can do while engaged in secular pursuits, under the influence of the unseen and eternal.

To the family, the Sabbatical institution is a blessing by promoting domestic order and education, family religion and affection.

It blesses the community by directly advancing intelligence, religion, and morality; and by indirectly securing the results of these—good legislation and social order.

Each of the topics treated in the preceding sections might have been indefinitely extended; and other topics might have been added; but as the main object throughout has been to show that the law of the Sabbath is founded in the constitution of man, it was deemed unnecessary to introduce any subject which did not directly contribute to this end.

This plan may seem to some to exclude the family and the state, or community, which have both received notice, in connection with the sacred day; but it really does not, for these institutions are natural and coeval with the human race. They are essential to the perpetuation and well-being of mankind, founded in the very necessities of our being, in a way that cannot be affirmed of other things that might have been introduced.

PART II.

SECTION I.

INSTITUTION OF THE SABBATH.

IF the law of the Sabbath is founded in the constitution of man, it seems to be a very obvious inference that it should be coeval with the human race. Being an institution of universal and permanent benefit, it must have had its origin among the first necessities of mankind.

But we are not left to *à priori* deduction on this point. After "the heavens and earth were finished, and all the host of them," God "rested on the seventh day from all his work which he had made. And God blessed the seventh day, and sanctified it: because that in it he had rested from all his work which God created and made." (Gen. ii. 2, 3.)

These verses clearly teach the paradisaical origin of the Sabbath as a day of holy rest and worship. What else can be inferred from God's blessing and sanctifying the seventh day, it is difficult to conceive. The Hebrew word, rendered in the English version, "sanctified," signifies in the Piel species, (the species used in Gen. ii. 3,) to make holy, to hallow, to regard and treat as holy, to consecrate. The language of the sacred writer, therefore, evidently means that the seventh day was consecrated, set apart to be a day of peculiar blessing to man. It was given to our first parents, at that time the whole human race; and the reason assigned for its institution is general, viz.: "God rested." As this reason is unlimited by locality or time, the institution cannot have reference to any particular people or to any particular age, but to every people and to every age.

The supposition that Moses had, in the passage quoted, anticipative reference to the fourth commandment, is unnatural, if the Sabbath is such an institution as we have endeavoured to show in the former part of this treatise. Being alike useful and important for mankind in general, in all ages, it would most naturally have its beginning when man commenced his existence. This view of its origin explains those intimations which sometimes appear in the book of Genesis, of the use of the number seven in designating periods of time.

1. A certain period of time is referred to in Gen. iv. 3, which is not said to have been the hebdomadal; but on the hypothesis that the Sabbath was previously instituted, scarcely a doubt can be entertained that the reference is to a weekly division.

2. Whatever uncertainty may exist in regard to the division of time alluded to above, there are passages which are sufficiently explicit. Noah observed the hebdomadal division of time. The

command was given to enter into the ark *seven* days before the flood came. (Gen. vii. 4, 10.) *Seven* days elapsed between the times of sending forth the dove. (Gen. viii. 10–12.) Jacob fulfilled a *week* (literally hebdomad,) for Rachel, (Gen. xxix. 27, 28;) and Joseph made a mourning for his father *seven* days. (Gen. l. 10.)

The next mention of the Sabbath is in Exodus xvi. 22–30. This was on the occasion of giving the manna, before the promulgation of the law from Mount Sinai. "And it came to pass," says the sacred historian, "that on the sixth day they gathered twice as much bread, two omers for one man: and all the rulers of the congregation came and told Moses. And he said unto them, This is that which the Lord hath said, To-morrow is the rest of the holy Sabbath unto the Lord: bake that which ye shall bake *to-day*, and seethe that ye will seethe; and that which remaineth over, lay up for you to be kept until the morning. And they laid it up till the morning as Moses bade; and it did not stink, neither was there any worm therein. And Moses said, Eat that to-day; for to-day is a Sabbath unto the Lord: to-day ye shall not find it in the field. Six days ye shall gather it; but on the seventh day, which is the Sabbath, there shall be none. And it came to pass, that there went out some of the people on the seventh day for to gather, and they found none. And the Lord said unto Moses, How long refuse ye to keep my commandments and my laws?

See, for that the Lord hath given you the Sabbath, therefore he giveth you on the sixth day the bread of two days: abide ye every man in his place, let no man go out of his place on the seventh day. So the people rested on the seventh day."

This passage speaks of the Sabbath as a thing known. Without naming it, or referring to it, God informed Moses that the Israelites should gather, on the sixth day, twice as much manna as on any other day. From this it would seem that the division of time, by weeks, was known when the Israelites went out of Egypt. This was before the giving of the law: therefore the obligation to observe the Sabbath is clearly enforced, irrespective of the Mosaic law.

The opening words of the fourth commandment —"Remember the Sabbath day"—imply that the institution was not a new one, though it had probably fallen into desuetude; and the reason assigned for its observance is a general one, and not connected with the deliverance of the Israelites from bondage.

The fact that some heathen nations, at a very early period, and some of a later date, observed a hebdomadal division of time, is an argument for the paradisaical origin of the Sabbath. We find traces of it, and of the Sabbatic principle, among the Phœnicians, Persians, Greeks, Romans, Slavonians, the natives of Pegu, the Chinese, the inhabitants of Guinea, and Mexicans. It is not probable that these nations derived it from the Jews, who were unknown to many of them, and hated by those to whom they were known. How, then, came they by it? Either the Sabbatic institution commended itself to their reason, or it was transmitted from one generation to another, from the very beginning of our race. If we accept the former hypothesis, it is in perfect harmony with the doctrine that the Sabbath is a natural institution, founded in our constitution; if the latter, it is in perfect harmony with the Bible account of its paradisaical origin.

An objection against the paradisaical origin of the Sabbath has been drawn from the silence of the Scriptures respecting its observance, until after the departure of the children of Israel from Egypt. It might as well be argued that it was not observed during the time of the judges, since there is no mention of the fact. But no one could be induced to believe, from the mere silence of the Scriptures on the subject, that an institution, which was re-enacted with so much solemnity at Sinai, and which was the key-note to a scale of Sabbatical observances among the Jews, had fallen into desuetude shortly after the death of Joshua. With as little probability, considering the frequent intimations of a hebdomadal division of time in the book of Genesis, can any one infer that it was not observed prior to the giving of the law. The silence of the Scriptures on the subject is not conclusive.

The duty of observing the Sabbath is sometimes

put upon a ground different from that given in the fourth commandment. "And the Lord spake unto Moses, saying, Speak thou also unto the children of Israel, saying, Verily my Sabbaths ye shall keep: for it is a sign between me and you throughout your generations; that ye may know that I am the Lord that doth sanctify you. Ye shall keep the Sabbath therefore; for it is holy unto you. Every one that defileth it shall surely be put to death: for whosoever doeth any work therein, that soul shall be cut off from among his people. Six days may work be done; but in the seventh is the Sabbath of rest, holy to the Lord: whosoever doeth any work in the Sabbath day, he shall surely be put to death. Wherefore the children of Israel shall keep the Sabbath, to observe the Sabbath throughout their generations, for a perpetual covenant. It is a sign between me and the children of Israel for ever: for in six days the Lord made heaven and earth, and on the seventh day he rested, and was refreshed." (Exodus xxxi. 12–17.) "And remember that thou wast a servant in the land of Egypt, and that the Lord thy God brought thee out thence through a mighty hand and by a stretched out arm; therefore the Lord thy God commanded thee to keep the Sabbath day." (Deut. v. 15.)

From these passages it may be clearly inferred that besides the re-enactment of the Sabbatical institution, at Sinai, there were special additions made to its observance, which belonged to the Jews only, and which were a part of their civil or ceremonial law. These additions were made for the reasons specified in the two passages that have been quoted:

1. As a sign of their covenant relation to the Lord. "Verily my Sabbath ye shall keep: for it is a sign between me and you throughout your generations; that ye may know that I am the Lord that doth sanctify you."

2. As a memorial of their deliverance from Egypt. "Remember that thou wast a servant in the land of Egypt, and that the Lord thy God brought thee out thence through a mighty hand and a stretched out arm: therefore the Lord thy God hath commanded thee to keep the Sabbath day."

With these ends in view the Sabbatical principle was extended to years, every seventh year being a year of rest. Moreover the violation of the Sabbath, among the Jews, was punished with death by the civil magistrate.

Since these things were for the Jews, as a nation, and hence designed for a particular purpose, and local in their nature, they ceased whenever that purpose was accomplished. They have passed away with the Jewish polity; while that which is moral and universal, that which "was made for man," and not for the Jews specially, remains, and will remain.

From this brief and imperfect discussion of the institution of the Sabbath we unhesitatingly conclude that its origin is coeval with that of man, for the following reasons:

1. The Sabbath being of universal and permanent benefit, and its law being founded in the constitution of man, must, one would suppose, be as old as the necessities which it is designed to supply. These necessities had their origin with our race.

2. The testimony of Scripture:

(*a*) The express mention of its institution, Gen. ii. 2, 3.

(*b*) Intimations, that appear in the book of Genesis, of the use of the number seven in designating periods of time, Gen. vii. 6–10; viii. 10–12; xxix. 27, 28; l. 10.

(*c*) The sacred narrative, Exodus xvi. 22–30.

(*d*) The opening words of the fourth commandment, and the fact that the reason assigned in that commandment for its observance is a general one.

3. The fact that some heathen nations, at a very early period, observed a hebdomadal division of time.

4. The fact that special reasons were given to the Jews for its observance leads us to infer that the general reason assigned in the fourth commandment was intended for all mankind; that it existed before the Jews were a nation, just as the rainbow may have existed before it was made the sign of the covenant with Noah.

5. We may add the fact that the fourth command-

ment is incorporated into a series of moral laws, which are universally binding, in all ages. These laws were not enacted, for the first time, at Sinai. From their very nature they must have existed from the origin of mankind. But the moral character of the Sabbath will form the subject of the next chapter.

SECTION II.

THE SABBATH A MORAL INSTITUTION.

Some take the ground that the Sabbath is a positive institution. Even Dr. Wayland, in his excellent work entitled "The Elements of Moral Science," says: "Although the Sabbath is a positive institution, and, therefore, the proof of its obligation is to be sought for entirely from revelation, yet there are indications in the present constitution, that periods of rest are necessary both for man and for beast." It is to be regretted that so eminent a man should have given his authority to such a doctrine. It is due to him, however, to say that his arguments on the subject agree better with the opposite doctrine, that the Sabbath is a moral institution.

But for the purpose of contributing to a clearer understanding of the matter, let us consider the distinction between *positive* and *moral*.

In the words of Bishop Butler, "Moral precepts are precepts the reasons of which we see; positive precepts are precepts the reasons of which we do not see. Moral duties arise out of the nature of the case itself, prior to external command. Positive duties do not arise out of the nature of the case, but from external command; nor would they be duties at all, were it not for such command received from Him whose creatures and subjects we are." (*Analogy*, part ii. chapter i.)

To place the subject in a still clearer light, a few illustrations may be useful.

The love of God, obedience to him, and obedience to parents are moral duties, because they arise from our relations to God and our parents. The reasons of them are seen. Hence the laws enjoining these duties are moral laws, binding upon the whole human race, at every period of its existence. The command to the Israelites to keep the Passover was positive, and the duty to observe it was positive, because prior to external command no reason could be seen for such an observance. Moral duties are commanded because they are right: positive duties are right because they are commanded.

We are now prepared to discuss the question whether the Sabbath is a positive or a moral institution.

1. The reason for the observance of the Sabbath existing in our constitution is deducible from the light of nature; and hence can be seen and felt prior to external command. This fact clearly shows the Sabbath to be a moral institution. The duties enjoined by it are such as are necessary to our well-

being as physical, intellectual, and moral creatures; and are not limited to any particular age, or nation, but are as enduring and universal as the human race. Experience confirms this statement. "Where the true religion has been unknown, it has always been found necessary to appoint, by some constituted authority, a certain number of holidays, which have often, even in heathen countries, exceeded, rarely anywhere have fallen short of, the number of God's instituted Sabbaths. The animal and mental, the bodily and spiritual natures of man alike demand them. Even Plato deemed the appointment of such days of so benign and gracious a tendency, that he ascribed them to that pity which the gods have for mankind born to painful labour, that they might have an ease and cessation from their toils. And what is this but an experimental testimony to the truth of God's having ordered his work of creation with a view to the appointment of such an institution in providence? and to his wisdom and goodness in having done so?" (Fairbairn's *Typology*, vol. ii. p. 116.)

2. The law enjoining the observance of the Sabbath is placed in the decalogue, which is acknowledged to be a summary of moral precepts. This is a testimony of the Divine Author of the decalogue to its moral character. Why did he place it among moral laws, written by his own hand, if it is merely positive? Why was the longest peal of the trumpet that which proclaimed the obligation

to "remember the Sabbath day to keep it holy," if it was a positive institution, designed to be merely temporary and local?

Observe, too, its position in the decalogue. It occupies a place intermediate to the commands of the first table and to those of the second, uniting the two tables, and securing, by its proper observance, the duties of both. In fact the duties of the Sabbath belong to both tables of the law, for they relate to the worship of God and to our own physical and moral culture.

The doctrine that the law of the Sabbath is moral, is in direct conflict with the opinion that it is a Jewish and temporary institution. The absurdity of such an opinion is, moreover, obvious from the very face of the fourth commandment. There is nothing in that commandment connected with individual interests, or national history. The great fact, on which it is based, is of equal significance to the world: it is universal in its bearing. "Thou shalt remember the Sabbath day to keep it holy, for in six days the Lord made heaven and earth, the sea and all that is in them, and rested on the seventh day." What is there here in the reason assigned for observing the seventh day, which is applicable to the Jews more than to any other people? Nothing. But abundant reason is given for its being kept sacred by all the creatures of God.

The conclusion at which we arrive from the fact that the law of the Sabbath is founded in the nature of man,—the reason for its observance being thus deducible from the light of nature—and from its position in a series of moral precepts, is that it is moral and not positive.

Notwithstanding this obvious conclusion, "it is argued by some, that whatever may have been the reason for admitting the law of the Sabbath into the ten commandments, and engraving it on tables of stone, it still is in its own nature different from all the rest. They are moral, and because moral, of universal force and obligation, while this is ceremonial, owing its existence to positive enactment, and, therefore, binding only so far as the enactment itself might be extended. The duties enjoined in the former are founded in the nature of things, and the essential relations in which men stand to God, or to their fellow-men; hence they do not depend on any positive enactment, but are co-extensive in their obligation with reason and conscience. But the law of the Sabbath, prescribing one day in seven to be a day of sacred rest, has its foundation simply in the authoritative appointment of God, and hence, unlike the rest, is not fixed and universal, but special and mutable."

The reasoning here cannot be admitted, for it has been shown that the Sabbatical institution is founded in the nature of things. It is founded in our constitution, and in the relations in which we stand to God. We require rest for both soul and body, and God must be worshipped; consequently some stated time should be set apart for these purposes. This the light of nature teaches.

But does it teach what proportion of time we should observe? whether a third, fourth, fifth, sixth, or seventh part of our weekly time? Or does it teach that we should observe the first day of the week in preference to the seventh? the fifth in preference to the sixth? The light of nature does not instruct us in regard to these things. Are not, then, the proportion of time and the day to be observed positive? It would seem so, if reason cannot determine them. What part, then, of the Sabbath is moral? Evidently the substance of it, or what may be called the Sabbatical institution. The form of it, that is, the proportion of time and the day, is positive. This conclusion is supported by the words of the fourth commandment, which does not say, remember the seventh day, (namely in order from the creation,) but "remember the Sabbath day, to keep it holy." So, in the end of the commandment, the words are not, the Lord blessed the seventh day; but "the Lord blessed the Sabbath day," (the Sabbatical institution,) "and hallowed it."

The Sabbath, therefore, considered as to its substance, is moral; and considered as to the proportion of time and the day of the week to be observed, it is positive. Uniting the substance and form, and characterizing the institution according to their respective natures, we may denominate it moral-positive.

Dr. Fairbairn, in his excellent work entitled, "The *Typology of Scripture*," (book iii. chap. ii. sec. 3,) makes some remarks on this subject, which seem neither clear nor satisfactory.

"It is true," says Dr. Fairbairn, "that the Sabbath is a positive institution, though intimately connected with God's work in creation; and apart from his high command, it could not have been ascertained by the light of reason, that one entire day should at regular intervals be consecrated for bodily and spiritual rest, and especially that one in seven was the proper period to be fixed upon. In this respect we can easily recognize a distinction between the law of the Sabbath, and the laws which prohibit such crimes as lying, theft, or murder. But it does not, therefore, follow, that the Sabbath is in such a sense a positive, as to be a merely partial, temporary, ceremonial institution, and like others of this description done away in Christ. For a law may be positive in its origin, and yet neither local nor transitory in its destination; it may be positive in its origin, and yet equally needed and designed for all nations and ages of the world.

"For of what nature, we ask, is the institution of marriage? The seventh commandment bears respect to that institution, and is thrown as a sacred fence around its sanctity. But is not marriage in its origin a positive institution? Has it any other foundation than the original act of God in making one man and one woman, and positively ordaining that the man should cleave to the woman, and the two be one flesh?"

Perhaps Dr. Fairbairn did not mean what these words seem to express. His error consists in not distinguishing between the substance of the Sabbath and its form. According to the principles on which he argues, every command of the decalogue, in its ultimate analysis, might be reduced to a positive precept. What "other foundation than the original act of God in making one man and one woman, and positively ordaining" that they should love and serve him, has the first, second, or third commandment? Is it said that its foundation is in our relation of creatures to God? That is true. But that relationship was constituted by the act of creation, which act depended upon the will of God. What foundation has the eighth commandment except the right of property? a right which has no existence prior to possession.

It is not necessary that the reasons of a moral precept should be absolute, or unconditioned, like the axioms of mathematics, but that they should grow out of the relations that God has constituted —relations that exist everywhere and through all time among those for whose direction and benefit the law is intended. That the reasons for the observance of the Sabbath grow out of such relations cannot be denied, if we consider its connection with our own physical and spiritual well-being and with the discharge of our duties to the Author of our being. In view of these, the light of reason teaches us the necessity of such an institution. It is, therefore, according to our definition, a moral institution. Observing the distinction between moral and positive already given, we cannot understand how "a law may be positive in its origin, and yet neither local nor transitory in its destination;" how "it may be positive in its origin, and yet equally needed and designed for all nations and ages of the world." If a positive law may be such, what is the distinction between positive and moral? Might not a positive law, according to Dr. Fairbairn, be discovered by the light of reason as well as a moral? The fact that a law is "equally needed and designed for all nations and ages of the world" is a clear proof that it is moral, inasmuch as it is founded on relations everywhere existing and perceived. Such a law is the Sabbath.

Dr. Fairbairn himself, in another paragraph of the same section, from which the quotation above is made, speaks as strongly and clearly on this point as any one would desire; with what consistency it is not easy to perceive.

"It deserves more notice, however," says Dr. Fairbairn, "than it usually receives in this point of view, and should alone be almost held conclusive, that the ground on which the obligation to keep the Sabbath is based in the command, is the most universal in its bearing that could possibly be conceived. 'Thou shalt remember the Sabbath-day to keep it holy, for in six days the Lord made heaven and earth, the sea and all that is in them, and rested on the seventh day.' There is manifestly nothing Jewish here; nothing connected with individual interests or national history; the grand fact, out of which the precept is made to grow, is of equal significance to the whole world; and why should not the precept be the same, of which it forms the basis? God's method of procedure in creating the visible heavens and earth, produced as a formal reason for instituting a distinctive, temporary Jewish ordinance. Could it be possible to conceive a more 'lame and impotent conclusion?' And this, too, in the most compact piece of legislation in existence! It seems, indeed, as if God, in the appointment of this law, had taken special precautions against the attempts which he foresaw would be made to get rid of the institution, and that on this account he laid its foundations first in the original framework and constitution of nature. The law, as a whole, and certain, also, of its precepts, he was pleased to enforce by considerations drawn from his dealings toward Israel, and the peculiar relations which he now holds to them. But when he comes to impose the obligation of the Sabbath, he rises far beyond any consideration of a special kind, or any passing event of history. He ascends to primeval time, and, standing as on the platform of the newly created world, dates from thence the commencement and the ordination of a perpetually recurring day of rest. Since the Lord has thus honoured the fourth commandment above the others, by laying for it a foundation so singularly broad and deep, is it yet to be held in its obligation and import the narrowest of them all? Shall this, strange to think, be the only one which did not utter a voice for all times and all generations?" (*Typology of Scripture*, book iii. chap. ii. sec. iii. pp. 111, 112, vol. ii.)

After using this language, how could Dr. Fairbairn say that the "Sabbath is a positive institution?" Can any words assert its moral character more strongly than the following? "The Lord has honoured the fourth commandment above the others, by laying for it a foundation singularly broad and deep."

SECTION III.

CHANGE OF THE SABBATH FROM THE SEVENTH DAY OF THE WEEK TO THE FIRST.

The morality of the Sabbath does not lie in observing the seventh day in order from the creation, or in observing any particular day of the week; but in observing such a seventh day, or such a proportion of time as God may determine and appoint. Hence the day, for important reasons, may be changed; and a great majority of Christians say that it has been changed from the seventh day of the week to the first.

"The seventh was an important day under the Mosaic economy, but various instances occur in which the eighth was honoured. Circumcision, a seal of the righteousness of the faith which Abraham had, yet being uncircumcised, was to be administered on the eighth day. On the eighth day were the first-born of the cattle to be offered to the Lord, and the sheaf of the first-fruits to be presented and accepted. On that day the consecration of Aaron and his sons, and the sanctification of the temple, were completed. These and similar transactions were shadows of things to come, but the body is of Christ. And where shall we find an eighth day signalized by any doings or blessings of Christ correspondent with the types except the day on which he rose from the dead? There is one typical representation in particular that calls for remark. It occurs in Ezekiel's vision of the temple. That this vision was not realized in the second temple appears from, besides other facts, the differences in its worship from that prescribed by the law of Moses; and that there will be no literal fulfilment of it at a future day, is obvious from several considerations, one of which is sufficient, and is, that sacrifice is for ever abolished by Christ, so that to attempt its revival would be to deny his sacrifice. The only supposable accomplishment of the vision is in the condition of the Christian church. And what is there that fulfils the following prediction, if not the first day of the week and its Christian worship? And when these days have expired, it shall be, that upon the *eighth day and so forward*, the priest shall make your burnt-offerings upon the altar, and your peace-offerings; and I will accept you, saith the Lord."—Ezekiel xliii. 27.—(*Gilfillan on the Sabbath*, p. 302.)

As the Sabbath, under the old economy, was the seventh day in order from the creation, the day specified by the prophet, in the passage quoted, must be the eighth in the same order, that is, the first day of the week.

We have then, in the Old Testament, an intimation that a change of day would be effected. Was the change made? We affirm that it was, on the ground of the following evidence:

1. After his resurrection from the dead, our Lord, who rose on the first day of the week, appeared to the eleven, who were gathered together in Jerusalem, on the same day. (Luke xxiv. 33–36.) On two other occasions, when the disciples were assembled, on the first day of the week, he appeared to them. (John xx. 19–26.)

2. The Holy Spirit was poured out on the day of Pentecost, which was the first day of the week. (Compare Num. xxviii. 26, with Levit. xxiii. 16.)

3. The Apostles and early Christians were accustomed to meet together for worship on the first day of the week. (Acts xx. 7; 1 Corinthians xvi. 2.)

From the first of these passages (Acts xx. 7,) it

is evident that the disciples met ordinarily upon the first day of the week for hearing the word and celebrating the sacrament of the Lord's supper; for it is not said that the apostle called them, but that they came together to break bread; and Paul, on this occasion, preached to them. Paul, moreover, abode with them seven days, as is evident from verse 6; and yet upon none of the seven days did they meet for the breaking of bread, except on the first day of the week; which is a clear proof that they held it for the Christian Sabbath.

The argument from 1 Cor. xvi. 2, is: That if collections for the poor are expressly commanded to be made on the first day of the week, it plainly follows that Christians must meet together on that day for this and other Sabbath services. That it was not a mere temporary precept, binding upon the church of Corinth only, is obvious from the context and from the introduction to the epistle, in which it is expressly affirmed that it was binding also upon the churches of Galatia; and that the epistle was not addressed to the church of Corinth only, but to "all that in every place call upon the name of Jesus Christ our Lord." (1 Cor. xvi. 1; 1 Cor. i. 2.)

4. In Rev. i. 10, the first day of the week is dignified with the title of the "Lord's Day."

That this was the first day of the week cannot be doubted, when we consider that no other day but the first can properly be called the Lord's Day, and that it was afterwards so styled by the early Christians.*

5. The first day of the week was observed by the primitive church as the Christian Sabbath.

Pliny remarks, in his letter to Trajan, that the Christians were accustomed, on a stated day, to meet before daylight, and repeat among themselves a hymn to Christ as to God, and to bind themselves, by a sacred obligation, not to commit any wickedness. That this stated day was the first day of the week, or the Lord's day, is evident from other testimony. Indeed, so well known was the custom of the early Christians on the subject, that the ordinary question put by their persecutors to the Christian martyrs, was, "Hast thou kept the Lord's day, *Dominicum servasti?*" To which the usual reply was, "I am a Christian. I cannot omit it." *Christianus sum; intermittere non possum.*

The Rev. Dr. Coleman says: "The principal season of public worship among the primitive Christians was the first day of the week. From the time of the apostles, it was customary for the disciples of Christ, both in town and country, to meet in some common accessible place on the return of that day. * * * The high and holy character the Christians of the primitive ages attached to it, is sufficiently indicated by their styling it the Lord's day; and from the glorious event of which it was

* The Westminster Assembly's Shorter Catechism, explained by way of Question and Answer.

the stated memorial, they hailed it as a weekly festival, on which no other sentiment was becoming or lawful but that of unbounded spiritual joy." (*Christian Antiquities*, p. 269.)

These statements are confirmed by the earliest ecclesiastical authorities. The author of the Epistle of Barnabas represents the Lord as speaking in this wise:

"The Sabbaths which you now keep are not acceptable to me; but those which I have made; when resting from all things I shall begin the eighth day, that is, the beginning of the other world." "Wherefore," the writer of the epistle adds, "we observe the eighth day with gladness, in which Jesus rose from the dead, and having been manifested, he ascended into heaven." (*Barnabæ Epistola* xv. p. 40, *Hefele's Patrum Apostolicorum Opera.*)

In the same testimony agree Justin Martyr, Ignatius, Athanasius, and Eusebius.

Abundant proof has been exhibited to show that by the example and authority of Christ and his apostles the Sabbath was changed from the seventh to the first day of the week.

The efficient cause of this change is the sovereign will of him, who is Lord of the Sabbath, and this will was intimated by his own example and by that of his inspired apostles. The moving cause was his resurrection from the dead. That glorious event was demonstrative evidence that he had finished the work of redemption, and therefore, the day of his resurrection was his resting day.

In view of the resurrection of Christ on the first day of the week, we see a propriety in making it the Christian Sabbath ever afterward; for God's rest in the work of creation was marred and spoiled by man's sin; but his rest in the work of redemption, entered into at the resurrection of Christ, is a rest in which he will have eternal and unchangeable pleasure. Besides, redemption being a far greater and more excellent work than creation—being a new creation—should be embalmed in our memories by the observance of that day which commemorates its completion. Our moral nature requires some such standing memorial. Does not this account for the fact that the Scriptures are so explicit in regard to the day of his resurrection, while they are silent as to the day of his birth? The latter was the beginning of his days of labour and sorrow; the former, of his victory and exaltation.

The change of the Sabbath from the seventh to the first day of the week is a return to the primeval day. The first *complete* day that Adam spent on earth was the Sabbath, which must have been to him the beginning of the week; and, on the supposition that the first six days were indefinite periods of time, as some geologists affirm, the computation of time by weeks must have commenced with it. But whether these days were indefinite periods, or twenty-four hours each, man's first day in the world was a Sabbath. Was there not a propriety, then, in commencing the new world—the world redeemed by Christ—with the Sabbath? Is it not a part of his "restitution of all things?"

SECTION IV.

THE PERPETUITY OF THE SABBATH.

The perpetuity of the Sabbath results from its moral character. Moral laws, as well as physical, which have their foundation in human nature, must, by reason of their very relation to that nature, continue as long as it continues. That nature, in all that is essential to its identity and personality, will exist for ever. Hence these laws, in their essential features, must have an equal duration. Given the relations out of which they arise, their existence will run parallel with that of the relations.

It is not necessary to recapitulate the proof that the law of the Sabbath is moral, occupying a place in a series of laws universally acknowledged to be such. But as it has been asserted by some men of high standing in the church, and of merited reputation, (Dr. McLeod and others of the established Church of Scotland,) that not only the fourth commandment, but the whole decalogue is abrogated, we trust a brief consideration of this point will not be considered irrelevant to our main design.

The reason assigned for the opinion that the Sabbath is abrogated is the preface of the decalogue,

"I am the Lord thy God, which have brought thee out of the land of Egypt, out of the house of bondage." This preface, say the abettors of that opinion, makes the decalogue a Jewish law, binding upon the Jews only. It was doubtless a special reason why they should obey the law of God; but it does not follow that other nations were thereby exempted from obedience. The argument stated logically would stand thus:

The Israelites were bound to obey the decalogue because God brought them out of Egypt. No other nation was brought by God out of Egypt. Therefore no other nation was bound to obey the decalogue.

The fallacy of the argument, to one acquainted with the structure of the syllogism, is obvious at the first glance. It is of the same nature with the following, the fallacy of which is evident to every one:

Such and such garden trees should produce fruit, on account of their careful culture. Such and such trees are not garden trees having careful culture. Therefore such and such trees should produce no fruit.

As well might one argue, because Paul says of Christians, "Ye are not your own, for ye are bought with a price; therefore, glorify God in your body and in your spirit, which are God's," therefore sinners are under no obligation to glorify God in the body and in the spirit.

The decalogue, as to its principles, and probably as to its form, is older than the Jewish nation. It was promulgated before the Lord descended upon Mount Sinai. The violation of it had been punished in the case of the first murderer. Moses himself was obliged to flee from Egypt because he had killed an Egyptian. The unconscious violation of the seventh commandment, on the part of Abimelech, king of Gerar, was punishèd by God long before he proclaimed from the top of the burning mountain, "Thou shalt not commit adultery."

This view is confirmed by the Jews themselves, who, it seems, had not vanity enough to claim the exclusive possession of the moral law. Their ancient commentators refer to what they called "the statutes of Adam," and at other times, "the precepts of the sons of Noah," which, according to the account of Maimonides, were substantially the same with the ten commandments. These commandments were republished from Mount Sinai, and a reason, adapted to the peculiar circumstances of the Israelites, assigned for their observance.

Hitherto it has been argued from the nature of moral laws, that they are permanent. Let us now adduce the testimony of their Author, and that of men whom he inspired to complete his revelation as to their perpetuity.

Christ says, in his sermon on the mount, "Think not that I am come to destroy the law, or the prophets. I am not come to destroy, but to fulfil." —Matt. v. 17.

It is not necessary for our purpose that we understand the word "law" in the passage as referring exclusively to the decalogue. We may include in it the moral, ceremonial, and civil law of the Jews, not the least part of which was destroyed, in its ultimate idea, by our Saviour, but carried out to its full ideal. He came to occupy "the throne of his father David," according to its ideal, to "reign over the house of Jacob"—the true Israel of God—"for ever." The ceremonial laws being typical of him and of his work, terminated in him, and of course could have no binding force after his expiation for sin and ascension to heaven. He fulfilled the ceremonial law by presenting himself as the reality, which it prefigured. But the moral law having nothing typical, or ceremonial, could not be thus fulfilled. It must have its fulfilment in a different way. Our Saviour came not to destroy, but to fulfil it. How, then, did he fulfil it? Hear his own explanation: "Ye have heard that it was said by them of old time, Thou shalt not kill, and whosoever shall kill shall be in danger of the judgment; but I say unto you, that whosoever is angry with his brother without a cause shall be in danger of the judgment, and whosoever shall say to his brother, Raca, shall be in danger of the council; but whosoever shall say, thou fool, shall be in danger of hell fire. * * * Ye have heard that it has been said by them of old time, Thou shalt not commit adultery, but I say unto you, that whosoever looketh on a woman to lust after her hath committed adultery with her already in his heart."

Can any exposition be clearer? He gave, in his teaching, to the moral law a breadth, a depth, and a comprehensiveness far exceeding the partial, superficial, and distorted views of the formalists of that age. Our Saviour taught that the law is spiritual, and that its meaning cannot be tied down to the mere letter of its prohibition. It extends to the thoughts and feelings. The man who is angry with his brother without a cause, is guilty; he who looks on a woman to lust after her has committed adultery in his heart. The righteousness of the followers of Christ must exceed that of the Scribes and Pharisees, which consisted in externals, if they would enter into the kingdom of heaven. If any of them "break one of these least commandments, and teach men so," they "shall be called the least in the kingdom of heaven, for till heaven and earth pass, one jot or one tittle shall in no wise pass from the law till all be fulfilled."

We might refer, in this connection, to our Saviour's answer to the inquiry of the rich young man, in which he makes no allusion to the ceremonial laws, but specifies several of the decalogue. It is clearly intimated in this reply that life would result from perfect obedience to the moral law, and that such was the original condition of life. Of course, then, the moral law was not Jewish in its origin, but it existed from the very first. It was the rule of man's obedience in the garden of Eden. When he fell, it was abrogated as a condition of life by means of the covenant of grace, but its claims still rested upon him until they were met by our Substitute upon the cross, when he "magnified the law and made it honourable." By his expiation our guilt was removed, by the gift of his Holy Spirit we are sanctified, brought into harmony with the law, and are enabled to "delight in it after the inward man." We do not make void the law through faith; yea, we establish the law.

In conformity with the teaching of our Saviour on this point, is that of his apostles.

Paul says: "Owe no man anything, but to love one another, for he that loveth another hath fulfilled the law. For this, Thou shalt not kill, Thou shalt not steal, Thou shalt not bear false witness, Thou shalt not covet, and if there be another commandment it is briefly comprehended in this saying: Thou shalt love thy neighbour as thyself. Love worketh no ill to his neighbour; therefore love is the fulfilling of the law." There is no doubt here as to the law Paul had in his mind, for he quotes some of its precepts, which he generalizes into one more comprehensive—"Thou shalt love thy neighbour as thyself." This is a law which shall never end; but it includes in it every precept of the second table, which must therefore remain. In the same way does the Apostle James speak of the moral law as being still in force: "If ye fulfil the royal law according to the scripture, Thou shalt love thy neighbour as thyself, ye do well; but if ye have respect to persons, ye commit sin, and are convinced of the law as transgressors. For whosoever shall keep the whole law, and yet offend in one point, he is guilty of all. For he that said, Do not commit adultery, said also, Do not kill. Now if thou commit no adultery, yet if thou kill, thou art become a transgressor of the law."

We may now, without hesitation, conclude, upon the authority of Christ and his apostles, that the decalogue was not abrogated with the ceremonial law. It is still in force. The teaching of Christ has given it a breadth, which was unknown, except, perhaps, to his inspired servants, before his incarnation. In this decalogue the law of the Sabbath is found. *It* is, therefore, still in force. "Remember the Sabbath day to keep it holy," still remains the hinge of the two tables of the moral law.

But does not Paul say: "One man esteemeth one day above another; another esteemeth every day alike. Let every man be fully persuaded in his own mind. He that regardeth the day regardeth it unto the Lord, and he that regardeth not the day, to the Lord he doth not regard it."—Rom. xiv. 5, 6.

And, "Ye observe days, and months, and times, and years. I am afraid of you, lest I have bestowed upon you labour in vain."—Gal. iv. 10, 11.

And "Let no man, therefore, judge you in meat or in drink, or of the Sabbath days."—Coloss. ii. 16.

An exegesis of these passages is not necessary to our purpose. It can easily be obtained in exegetical works (such as Hodge's and Ellicott's) on Paul's epistles. That there is no reference to the Christian Sabbath is evident for the following reasons:

1. Paul is speaking of Jewish festivals. His argument and the context are not consistent with any other exposition.

2. Paul himself observed the Christian Sabbath, (Acts xx. 7,) and enjoined upon Christians to perform a certain duty on that day, which duty, we have seen, was neither temporary nor local. See page 61.

3. The early Christians observed the Christian Sabbath, (pp. 61, 62,) and between them and Paul, so far as negative testimony is worth anything, there existed no difference of opinion.

4. Paul acknowledges the binding authority of the moral law, in which the law of the Sabbath is included.

5. The ten commandments were written by the hand of God on tables of stone, to indicate their durability, and no intimation was ever given that the fourth would be erased.

6. It is distinctly stated, in Deut. x. 4, that there are ten commandments, which would not be true if the fourth is abrogated.

7. Isaiah, referring to the present dispensation,

(lvi. 2,) says: "Blessed is the man that keepeth the Sabbath from polluting it."

But, it may be asked, if the law of the Sabbath is not abrogated, why is there not more explicit mention in the New Testament of the duty of observing it? For the reason that there was no necessity for such mention. Its law was found in a moral code which is of perpetual obligation.

SECTION V.

SUMMARY.

We have endeavoured to show—with what success we will leave others to judge—that the Sabbath was instituted in Paradise; that it is, as to its substance, a *moral* institution, and as to its substance and form a *moral-positive* institution; that it has been changed from the seventh day of the week to the first; and that it is perpetual.

These positions, if they have been successfully maintained, are directly antagonistic to and subversive of the following errors, viz: That the Sabbath is a Jewish institution, having no existence before the promulgation of the law from Mount Sinai; that it has passed away with the Mosaic economy; that its law is positive and not moral; and that the seventh day of the week is the divinely authorized, immutable Sabbath.

The facts of its institution and perpetuity are also subversive of the opinion of those who hold all days to be alike common, or alike sacred. If the Lord has "blessed the Sabbath day, and hallowed it," and allowed us six days for our own employments, then all days are not alike common, or alike sacred. One day in seven is more sacred than the other six, because it is the Lord's day consecrated to his service and to the benefit of man. This doctrine, that one day in seven is holy to the Lord, by his own appointment, is utterly at variance with the opinion that the claims of the Sabbath are satisfied by the observance of certain canonical hours. The whole day must be kept sacred. God blessed the *Sabbath day*, not a few hours.

PART III.

THE SANCTIFICATION OF THE SABBATH.

SECTION I.

PRELIMINARY OBSERVATIONS.

IN the record of the original institution of the Sabbath we read that "God blessed the seventh day and sanctified it," and in the fourth commandment it is said, "the Lord blessed the Sabbath day and hallowed it."

God's blessing the seventh day—the Sabbath day in the fourth commandment—means that he made a distinction between it and other days. He made it a source of peculiar blessings to man. His sanctifying it signifies that he set it apart from a common to a religious use.

That which is set apart for such a use, is the day, not a few canonical hours. "God blessed the seventh *day* and sanctified it." Like other days the Sabbath is measured by one revolution of the earth on its axis.

The reasons assigned in the fourth commandment for our remembering the Sabbath day to keep it holy, are:

1. God's challenging a special property in the Sabbath day. "The seventh day is the Sabbath of the Lord thy God."

2. His example. "In six days the Lord made heaven and earth, the sea, and all that in them is, and rested the seventh day."

3. His blessing the Sabbath day and hallowing it. "Wherefore the Lord blessed the Sabbath day, and hallowed it."

4. In addition to these expressed reasons there is an implied reason, viz. That having six days of the week for our own employment, we would be both unreasonable and ungrateful, if we refused to devote a seventh part of our time to the more immediate service and worship of God.

No other commandment of the decalogue has so many reasons expressed and implied for its observance, as the fourth. This is itself a proof of the great importance that God attaches to the sanctification of the Sabbath. It is also an implication of the proneness of men to desecrate the holy day, and it renders the violation of it the more inexcusable.

The reasons for keeping holy the Sabbath day being so numerous and so cogent, the question arises, "How is the Sabbath to be sanctified?" The answer contained in our Shorter Catechism is full and explicit: "The Sabbath is to be sanctified by a holy resting all that day, even from such worldly employments and recreations as are lawful on other days, and spending the whole time in the public and private exercises of God's worship, except so much as is to be taken up in the works of necessity and mercy."

We are here taught:

1. That the Sabbath is to be sanctified by a holy resting all that day. Exod. xx. 10—"In it thou *shalt* not do any work." See, also, Exod. xxxi. 15; Deut. v. 14; Lev. xxiii. 3.

2. That we are to abstain from all worldly employments on the Sabbath. Jer. xvii. 21—"Thus saith the Lord, Take heed to yourselves, and bear no burden on the Sabbath day." See, also, Neh. xiii. 15, 16–22; Luke xxiii. 56.

3. That we are to abstain from recreations and pastimes on the Sabbath, although lawful on other days. Is. lviii. 13—"If thou turn away thy foot from the Sabbath, from doing thy pleasure on my holy day, and call the Sabbath a delight, the holy of the Lord, honourable; and shalt honour him, not doing thine own ways, nor finding thine own pleasure, nor speaking thine own words."

4. That the Sabbath is to be employed in the public exercises of God's worship. Isa. lxvi. 23—"From one Sabbath to another shall all flesh come to worship before me, saith the Lord."

5. That the Sabbath is to be employed in private acts of secret and social worship. Lev. xxiii. 3—"It is the Sabbath of the Lord in all your dwellings." See, also, Ps. xcii. title.

6. That works of necessity are lawful on the Sabbath day. Matt. xii. 1—"Jesus went on the Sabbath day through the corn; and his disciples were an hungered and began to pluck the ears of corn and to eat." See, also, ver. 2–8.

7. That works of mercy are lawful on the Sabbath day. Luke xiii. 16—"Ought not this woman, being a daughter of Abraham, whom Satan hath bound, lo, these eighteen years, to be loosed from this bond on the Sabbath day?" See, also, Matt. xii. 9–13.—*Peterson on the Shorter Catechism*, pp. 204, 205.

These directions are plain, and supported by Scriptural authority. But in order to answer the question, How is the Sabbath to be sanctified? rightly, we must keep distinctly before us the objects of the Sabbath. These are to perpetuate the knowledge and worship of Jehovah, to promote the spiritual, moral, and physical welfare of men. How must the day be kept, in order most fully to promote these objects? The answer to this question now claims our attention.

SECTION II.

THE SABBATH IS TO BE KEPT IN SUCH A WAY AS TO PERPETUATE THE KNOWLEDGE AND WORSHIP OF JEHOVAH.

The intimate connection between the sanctification of the Sabbath and the preservation of the knowledge of God is plainly intimated in Exodus xxxi.

13: "Speak thou also unto the children of Israel, saying, Verily my Sabbaths ye shall keep, for it is a sign between me and you throughout your generations, that ye may know that I am the Lord that doth sanctify you."

This knowledge is the most important that we can possess. "This is life eternal, that they might know thee the only true God, and Jesus Christ whom thou hast sent."—John xvii. 3. "For this is the covenant that I will make with the house of Israel after those days, saith the Lord, I will put my laws into their minds, and write them in their hearts; and I will be to them a God, and they shall be to me a people. And they shall not teach every man his neighbour, and every man his brother, saying, Know the Lord; for all shall know me from the least to the greatest."—Heb. viii. 10, 11.

To reveal this knowledge clearly and fully, the Eternal Word became incarnate. "No man hath seen God at any time; the only begotten Son, which is in the bosom of the Father, he hath declared him."—John i. 18. "In him was life, and the life was the light of men."—John i. 4.

To preserve and propagate this knowledge is the duty of the church. "Go ye into all the world and preach the gospel to every creature."—Mark xvi. 15. "Ye are the light of the world. * * * Let your light so shine before men, that they may see your good works and glorify your Father which is in heaven."—Matt. v. 14, 16. "Among whom ye shine as lights in the world; holding forth the word of life."—Phil. ii. 15, 16.

To receive this knowledge and to be guided by it is the duty of all men. "How long, ye simple ones, will ye love simplicity? and the scorners delight in their scorning, and fools hate knowledge? Turn ye at my reproof; behold, I will pour out my Spirit unto you, I will make known my words unto you."—Prov. i. 22, 23. "Get wisdom, get understanding; forget it not, neither decline from the words of my mouth."—Prov. iv. 5.

For instruction in this knowledge the Sabbath has been graciously given to us. It is called "the Sabbath of the Lord thy God;" his day in a special sense, set apart for his worship and the preservation of the true religion. For this end it ought to be observed. How must we observe it to secure this end?

1. By the diligent and prayerful reading and study of God's holy word, the only infallible source of divine knowledge.

Amidst the multiplicity of religious books, papers, and periodicals, the Bible is sadly neglected by Christians of the present day. For this reason they have defective views of divine truth, possessing no clear conception of the doctrines that they profess to believe, and in too many instances but a feeble conviction of their importance, consequently they are weak and stunted in spiritual frame and stature, and do not attain to the thew and vigour of the

Bible-reading Christians of the seventeenth century. How applicable to the great majority of Christians of this generation are the words of Paul to the Hebrews: "For when for the time ye ought to be teachers, ye have need that one teach you again which be the first principles of the oracles of God, and are become such as have need of milk, and not of strong meat."—Heb. v. 12. In this state of spiritual infancy they must continue as long as they neglect the careful reading and diligent study of the Scripture, which "is profitable for doctrine, for reproof, for correction, for instruction in righteousness, that the man of God may be perfect, thoroughly furnished unto all good works."—2 Tim. iii. 16. Let such, then, as desire to grow in divine knowledge and grace, peruse daily the pages of God's holy word, let them make it especially their Sabbath book, searching in its inexhaustible mines for those riches that endure for ever, seeking from its spiritual storehouses the aliment of the soul. Oh that men would prize more this

"Most wondrous book! bright candle of the Lord!
Star of eternity! the only star
By which the bark of man could navigate
The sea of life, and gain the coast of bliss
Securely; only star which rose on Time,
And on its dark and troubled billows still,
As generation, drifting swiftly by,
Succeeded generation, threw a ray
Of heaven's own light, and to the hills of God,
The everlasting hills, pointed the sinner's eye."

2. We must observe the Sabbath by a punctual, serious, and prayerful attendance upon the institutions and ordinances of Christ's appointment.

The great institution which Christ has appointed for the instruction of mankind in religion and morals, is the church, and the divinely ordained ordinances which she employs for this purpose are the preaching of the word, the sacraments and prayer.

Of these ordinances Protestants are accustomed to assign the first place to preaching. It is certainly the most important, but the others are by no means to be neglected. "The preacher goes forth as a messenger of the King of kings to announce to a lost world the tidings of salvation through a risen Saviour. He proclaims the one only name given under heaven, or among men, whereby they must be saved. He cries aloud and spares not. He urgently entreats and fervently beseeches men, as in Christ's stead, to be reconciled to God. And to leave them without excuse, he reasons of temperance, righteousness, and a judgment to come."

Differing from every other system of human teaching, and rising in its objects superior to any unaided conceptions of the human mind, preaching aims at the eternal salvation of the souls of men. This aim embraces two important elements:

The conversion of men from error and sin.

Their instruction and edification in Christian truth.

"Here are objects involving everything of most importance to the welfare of the life that now is, and of that which is to come; objects, moreover, of universal necessity. There is no condition of humanity that does not demand the preaching of the gospel. There is no nation it may not exalt. There is no soul that does not crave the blessing it proposes to confer. Yet no other agency is so adapted to secure that blessing. Philosophy fails, learning falls short, and human power is insufficient. But the preaching of the Cross proves to be the power of God unto salvation, to the Jews first, and also to the Gentiles."—Kidder's *Homiletics*, pp. 30, 31.

The sacraments represent to our senses what the word represents to our faith. They exhibit to us, by means of symbols, the great facts of redemption, and are admirably fitted to keep alive a knowledge of these facts in the world.

By social prayer we acknowledge, as it is meet that we should, all our social and civil blessings to be the gift of God. This is one of the most important duties of the Sabbath day, and ought to be duly observed.

3. To these public and social exercises of religion may be added the instruction of the young in Sabbath schools and in the family, the importance of which to the highest interests of the church cannot be overestimated. Indeed, the religious training of the young forms an important part of the duty

of every pastor and of every Christian parent. It cannot be omitted without great injury to the church. The children of believers are the hope of the church. It is to them chiefly that it must look for increase. Hence it ought to feel the greatest solicitude that they be brought "up in the nurture and admonition of the Lord."

By the observance of these ordinances the knowledge of God and the true religion are preserved in the world. But without the Sabbath it would be impossible to preserve these ordinances themselves; hence the necessity of devoting part of it to the public exercises of God's worship and to the teaching of religion. This is the principal end of the Sabbath; consequently those who do not consecrate part of it to this, use their influence to banish the knowledge of God and religion from the earth.

SECTION III.

THE SABBATH IS TO BE SANCTIFIED BY ATTENDING TO THE PRIVATE EXERCISES OF RELIGION.

Under the private exercises of religion are comprehended secret and family religious duties. Secret duties are secret prayer, reading the Scriptures by one's self, and other religious books of a devotional and practical character; meditation upon divine things and self-examination. The religious duties of the family are family worship, family catechizing and conference.

Without these private and family exercises of religion the public ordinances of the sanctuary would be of little avail. The mind and heart of the hearer would be in a condition unfavourable to the reception of the preached word and out of harmony with the solemn duties of the house of God. He could not adopt the language of the Psalmist: "As the hart panteth after the water brooks, so panteth my soul after thee, O God. My soul thirsteth for God, for the living God: when shall I come and appear before God?" Ps. xlii. 1, 2. "How amiable are thy tabernacles, O Lord of hosts! My soul longeth, yea, even fainteth for the courts of the Lord: my heart and my flesh crieth out for the living God." Ps. lxxxiv. 1, 2. It is in the hours of private devotion, when the joys of salvation fill his heart, that the Christian can say: "One thing have I desired of the Lord, that will I seek after; that I may dwell in the house of the Lord all the days of my life, to behold the beauty of the Lord, and to inquire in his temple." Ps. xxvii. 4.

On the other hand, the services of the sanctuary fit the Christian for the duties of the closet, just as conversation fits a man for solitude. If he has been a diligent and devout hearer, he carries home with him food for the soul. Subjects for meditation and prayer have been suggested to him; and motives for increased activity and zeal have been presented to his mind. Thus the public and private exercises of religion act and react upon one another, the one forming a preparation for the other.

The cause of the dwarfish spiritual stature of so many Christians may be found in their neglect of private, personal religion on the holy Sabbath. They may plead some excuse for such neglect on other days, when they are engaged in secular affairs; but they cannot find any excuse on the Lord's day. One of its main objects is to promote the spiritual interests of man; and if we do not employ it for that purpose, we do not use it in conformity with its design. Were it more faithfully spent in reading God's holy word, in self-examination; in prayer for deeper repentance, for stronger faith, for a brighter hope, for growth in all the graces of the Spirit, for strength to discharge our duty, for a blessing upon the public ordinances of the sanctuary, for the triumph of Christ's kingdom, we would not find so many that are weak and sickly among us, so many that sleep. We would not hear so frequently the mournful complaint:

"What peaceful hours I once enjoyed!
How sweet their memory still!
But they have left an aching void,
The world can never fill."

But Christians would be strengthened with might by the Spirit in the inner man; Christ would dwell in their hearts by faith; they would be rooted and grounded in love, "able to comprehend with all saints what is the breadth, and length, and depth, and height, and to know the love of Christ, which passeth knowledge." Eph. iii. 16–19. Their song would be:

"The men of grace have found
Glory begun below;
Celestial fruits on earthly ground,
From faith and hope may grow.

"The hill of Zion yields
A thousand sacred sweets,
Before we reach the heavenly fields,
Or walk the golden streets.

"Then let our songs abound,
And every tear be dry;
We're marching through Immanuel's ground,
To fairer worlds on high."

Not less important than the private exercises of religion are the religious duties of the family on the Sabbath. These, we have already stated, are family worship and catechizing, together with religious conference. It is certainly eminently fit and becoming for all that are united in the domestic relation, or who are dwelling in the same house and family, to join in singing God's praise, in reading his word, in studying its doctrines, in applying them, and in praying to their Father in heaven. Besides the propriety of such exercises, there is express warrant for them in the word of God. The commandments, the statutes, and the judgments which the Lord commanded the Israelites, they were commanded to teach diligently unto their children, to talk of them when sitting in their houses, when walking by the way, when lying down, and when rising up. Deut. vi. 7. Men are exhorted to pray everywhere with all prayer and supplication; surely then and by necessary consequence in the family. Eph. vi. 18; 1 Tim. ii. 8. And the prophet prays to Jehovah to pour his fury upon the heathen that do not know him and upon the families that call not on his name. Jer. x. 25.

We have, moreover, examples of family religion recorded in Scripture for our imitation. Abraham commanded his children and his household after him, that they should keep the way of the Lord, to do justice and judgment. Gen. xviii. 19. Joshua resolved for himself and his house to serve the Lord. Josh. xxiv. 15. David blessed his household. 2 Sam. vi. 20. Cornelius feared God with all his house. Acts x. 2.

In view of these precepts and examples are not Christian families, who neglect family religion, greatly remiss in duty? How can they expect the blessing of Him who has enjoined upon parents to teach diligently unto their children his commandments, his statutes, and his judgments? This duty cannot be delegated to Sabbath-schools. They were never designed to supersede family instruction, though, in many instances they have done so. They should be used merely as auxiliaries: the parents should be the teachers and guides of their household, and for the performance of this duty God will hold them responsible.

The discharge of this duty is a constant thing. Children are to be trained up, brought up from childhood, in the nurture and admonition of the Lord. Eph. vi. 4. This does not hinder, but rather falls in with their special training on special occasions. No occasion can be so favourable to special religious instruction and training as the Sabbath, which we are commanded to observe in all our dwellings. Levit. xxiii. 3.

SECTION IV.

THE SABBATH IS TO BE SANCTIFIED BY BODILY REST, AND BY INTERMITTING SUCH INTELLECTUAL EMPLOYMENTS AS ARE NOT IMMEDIATELY CONNECTED WITH THE SERVICES OF RELIGION.

The advantages of the Sabbath as a day of rest have been already considered. In confirmation of these advantages we quoted the testimony of the late John Richard Farre, M. D., of London, before the British House of Commons, with reference to the effects of labouring seven days in the week, compared with those of labouring only six and resting one. We will repeat part of that testimony and make an additional quotation:

"As a day of rest," says the Doctor, "I view it [the Sabbath] as a day of compensation for the inadequate restorative power of the body under continued labour and excitement. * *

* * * * *

I consider, therefore, that in the bountiful provision of Providence for the preservation of human life, the Sabbatical appointment is not, as it has been sometimes theologically viewed, simply a precept partaking of a political institution, but that it is to be numbered among the natural duties, if the preservation of life be admitted to be a duty, and the premature destruction of it to be a suicidal act." —*Sabbath Manual*, pp. 35, 36.

Admitting the preservation of life to be a duty and its premature destruction to be a suicidal act, the Sabbath ought to be observed in such a way as to preserve life and prevent premature destruction, by making it a day of compensation for the "inadequate restorative power of the body under continued labour and excitement." For this end we must abstain from all bodily labour, except such as works of necessity, mercy, and piety require, and seek such a measure of physical rest as is consistent with the faithful discharge of the private and public duties of religion. Of that measure, each man's conscience, enlightened by the word of God, must be the judge.

In strict conformity with the physiological reasons for resting on the Sabbath is the Divine commandment, which requires us to cease from labour on that holy day, even in earing-time and in harvest —seasons when labour is most urgent.

The command applies to the mind as well as to the body. Those who are engaged in intellectual pursuits require periodical relaxation as well as those who are employed in manual labour. If they do not avail themselves of it, their minds soon lose their vigour and elasticity, and sink into premature decay. Besides, the duties of religion render it necessary to interrupt the regular routine of thought for the contemplation of spiritual things. These refresh the wearied mind as the waters of the fountain refresh the thirsty traveller in the desert.

The effects of both bodily and mental labour on the Sabbath may be seen in some ministers of religion, whose arduous duties do not allow them, as they think, any relaxation to recover their exhausted energies. Engrossed, during the week, in parochial duties and in preparation for the pulpit, obliged, sick or well, to preach twice every Sabbath, failure of health and temporary retirement from the active duties of the ministry, if not complete exhaustion and premature death, must be the necessary result. To prevent this it is necessary for them to enjoy, during the week, an equivalent for the Sabbath, on which the duties of their vocation call them to labour. With this periodical rest their health will be preserved, their term of life prolonged, and their usefulness increased.

Some advocate for those who have been confined

at hard labour during the week, especially in factories, the opening of art-galleries, the frequenting of beer-gardens, and pleasure excursions on the Sabbath. It is argued that such things, and the fresh air and scenery of the country, contribute to cheerfulness and health. Others, perceiving the incongruity between the sanctity of the Sabbath and such amusements, apologize for them, on the ground that if the labouring masses do not indulge in them they will indulge in something worse. It is merely a choice between two evils—a greater and a less. The former ignore the religious obligation to observe the Sabbath; the latter, admitting it, and assuming that it must be violated in one way or other, think that it is better to violate it decently than indecently.

No man, who has a right understanding of the ends for which the Sabbath was instituted, can, for a moment, countenance such views. The spiritual ends of the Sabbath are the first and most important; its physiological and sanitary ends are secondary and subordinate. The first transcend the second as far as the soul transcends the body. Being an institution principally designed for preserving the knowledge of God and the true religion in the world, and for the special culture of man's spiritual nature, it ought to be observed in such a way as best to secure these objects. That this can be best done by pleasure excursions, picture-galleries, public amusements and beer-gardens, would require a considerable degree of audacity to assert. Moreover, cheerfulness is best promoted by obedience to the laws of our spiritual and moral nature; and as the laws of the body never conflict with these laws, the pursuit of health is always consistent with the highest interests of our being.

The instances of best health and longevity, other things being equal, are among those who walk in the path of the Divine commandments, in the keeping of which there is great reward. The wicked do not live out half their days; for, as a general thing, the violation of the laws of our moral being carries along with it the violation of the laws of our physical being. In perfect obedience to moral law, therefore, do we find perfect safety and perfect harmony. All the elements of our highest development, both physical and spiritual, meet in doing the will of God.

SECTION V.

THE DUTY OF THE STATE WITH REFERENCE TO THE SANCTIFICATION OF THE SABBATH.

"How far any government has a right to interfere in matters touching religion has been a subject much discussed by writers upon public and political law. The right and the duty of the interference of government in matters of religion have been maintained by many distinguished authors, as well by those who were the warmest advocates of free governments as by those who were attached to governments of a more arbitrary character. Indeed, the right of a society or government to interfere in matters of religion will hardly be contested by any person who believes that piety, religion, and morality are intimately connected with the well-being of the state, and indispensable to the administration of civil justice. The promulgation of the great doctrines of religion, the being, and attributes, and providence of one Almighty God; the responsibility to him for all our actions, founded upon moral accountability; a future state of rewards and punishments; the cultivation of all the personal, social, and benevolent virtues;—these never can be a matter of indifference in any well-ordered community. It is, indeed, difficult to conceive how any civilized society can well exist without them. And, at all events, it is impossible for those who believe in the truth of Christianity, as a Divine revelation, to doubt that it is the especial duty of government to foster and encourage it among all the citizens and subjects. This is a point wholly distinct from that of the right of private judgment in matters of religion, and of the freedom of public worship according to the dictates of conscience.

"The real difficulty lies in ascertaining the limits to which government may rightfully go in fostering and encouraging religion. Three cases may easily be supposed: One where a government affords aid to a particular religion, leaving all persons free to adopt any other; another, where it creates an ecclesiastical establishment for the propagation of the doctrines of a particular sect of that religion, leaving a like freedom to all others; and a third, where it creates such an establishment, and excludes all persons not belonging to it, either wholly or in part, from any participation in the public honours, trusts, emoluments, privileges, and immunities of the state. For instance, a government may simply declare that the Christian religion shall be the religion of the state, and shall be aided and encouraged in all the varieties of sects belonging to it; or, it may declare that the Roman Catholic or Protestant religion shall be the religion of the state, leaving every man to the free enjoyment of his own religious opinions; or, it may establish the doctrines of a particular sect, as exclusively the religion of the state, tolerating others to a limited extent, or excluding all not belonging to it from all public honours, trusts, emoluments, privileges, and immunities.

"Probably, at the adoption of the Constitution, and of the amendment to it now under consideration, the general, if not the universal, sentiment in America was, that Christianity ought to receive encouragement from the state, so far as such encouragement was not incompatible with the private rights of conscience and the freedom of religious worship. An attempt to level all religions, and to make it a matter of state policy to hold all in utter indifference, would have created universal disapprobation, if not universal indignation." (*Familiar Exposition of the Constitution of the United States,* by Joseph Story, LL.D., pp. 260, 261.)

"Chancellor Kent declares that the Constitution of the State of New York never meant to withdraw religion in general, and with it the best sanctions of moral and social obligation, from all consideration and notice of the law."

"When Chief Justice of the Supreme Court, he used this language: 'No government among any of the polished nations of antiquity, and none of the institutions of modern Europe, (a single and monitory case excepted,) ever hazarded such a bold experiment upon the solidity of the public morals, as to permit with impunity, and under the sanction of their tribunals, the general religion of the community to be openly insulted and defamed. The very idea of jurisprudence with the ancient lawgivers and philosophers embraced the religion of the country.' So, he argues, it can be no less with us, for we are a Christian people, and the morality of the country is deeply engrafted upon Christianity." (*The Hebrew Lawgiver,* by Rev. J. M. Lowrie, D. D., vol. ii., pp. 56, 57.)

To the same purport might be quoted the opinions of many other celebrated jurists.

These views are sound and judicious. Religion can never be a matter of indifference in any well-ordered community. It is essential to the well-being of a state, and, consequently, its institutions should be honoured and protected by civil authority. The Divine justice being the ground of human law, all legislation should proceed upon the belief of the "being, attributes, and providence of one Almighty God; of our responsibility to him for all our actions;" and of "a future state of rewards and punishments;" and whatever tends to weaken this belief should be reprobated. "The fairest and most excellent preamble to all laws," says Plato, "is, that the gods not only *are*, but that they are also good, and that, moreover, they have an esteem for justice beyond anything that is felt among men." "That such views," says Cicero, "are useful and necessary, who will deny, when he reflects how many things must be confirmed by an oath, how much safety there is in those religious rites that pertain to the solemnization of contracts, how many the fear of Divine punishment keeps back from crime; in short, how sacred and holy a thing society becomes when the immortal gods are constantly presented (in the law) both as judges and witnesses." (*Plato against the Atheists,* Tayler Lewis's edition, pp. 110, 111.)

Obedience to moral law, whether on the part of the state or of the individual, is the only condition of safety. Every violation brings a recoil, which is prophetic of final destruction. The process of destruction, at first, may be slow and scarcely perceptible; but every step will prepare for another with accelerated speed, until ruin will come upon the wings of the whirlwind. Then repentance will be in vain: the transgressor will reap a harvest of woe. That this is the doom of both individuals and nations that continue in the transgression of God's law, both his word and providence give ample confirmation. It should, then, be esteemed a matter of the highest moment, in every well-ordered community, to protect, by every proper means, the Divine law from infraction, and to foster the institutions of religion as the only sure and effectual means of promoting social prosperity and happiness. The state, of course, cannot enforce religious duties, which, if acceptably performed, must be voluntary; but it can remove all hinderances to the performance of them, and afford that encouragement to the discharge of them which their permanent importance and beneficent influence deserve.

Not only has the state power to do this, but it is its duty to do it—a duty which fidelity to its trust requires it to discharge. But would not the state, in this case, intrude on the province of religion? Would it not practically unite the ecclesiastical and the civil? We may ask, in turn, is the state absolved from all religious obligation? Is the state atheistic? or is it, at best, deistic? Very few, except atheists and infidels would answer in the affirmative.

But the true ground on which to base Sabbath legislation, on the part of the state, is, in my opinion, that the Sabbath is not only a *religious*, but also a *natural* institution. Its law has its foundation in our physical, intellectual, and moral constitution; and consequently the observance of that law is necessary to bodily health, good order, and public morals. Obedience to it is obedience to the law of our nature. As such—as a natural institution—the state has a perfect right to enjoin the observance of the Sabbath, and to punish the violation of it as dangerous to the best interests of society. Omitting this, it fails in duty.

It is acknowledged by all that the state has the power, and that it is its duty to enact and enforce sanitary measures; to found educational establishments; to foster and protect every thing that has for its object the moral, intellectual, and social elevation of the people. It is not enough for the state to punish crime: it ought to devise and put in operation means and agencies to prevent it. What better preventive can be devised than a sober and decent observance of the Sabbath? What institution tends so much to promote all that is beautiful and orderly in domestic and social life? What tends more to preserve health, to prolong life, to encourage industry, and cultivate every moral virtue? Statistics have already been quoted to show that men who observe the Sabbath as a day of rest are more healthy, more moral, more orderly, and perform more work, than those who spend it in labour. Still greater is the contrast between those who "rest according to the commandment," and those who make it a day of amusement and dissipation. By the latter, released from their usual employments, it is made an occasion of debauchery and drunkenness. It would be better for the public and for themselves if they were compelled to work during the whole week. This assertion is fully sustained by the operation of the "Sunday Clause in the Excise Law" of New York. This clause reads as follows:

"All persons as herein provided shall keep the places at which they are so licensed to keep, sell, give, and dispose of strong and spirituous liquors, wines, ale, and beer, orderly and quiet, and between the hours of twelve o'clock at night and sunrise, and on *Sundays, completely and effectually closed.* Nothing herein contained shall be construed to prevent hotels from receiving and otherwise entertaining the travelling public upon Sundays, subject to the restrictions contained in this section."

Under the operation of this clause, the following results have been obtained.

Number of arrests for intoxication and disorderly conduct:	
On three Sundays in January 1866, under the old system	266
On three Sundays in January 1867, under the new law.	130
Net reduction	136
On four Sundays in February 1866, under the old system	402
On four Sundays in February 1867, under the new law.	320
Net reduction	82

On four Sundays in March 1866, under the old system..	474
On four Sundays in March 1867, under the new law......	258
Net reduction..	216
On four Sundays in April 1866, under the old system....	584
On four Sundays in April 1867, under the new system...	300
Net reduction..	284
Total reduction on 15 Sundays in 1867..................	718

"The Metropolitan Police authorities declare that, during the same period, their work on Sunday has been diminished one half. Nor is this all. The decrease of drunkenness and crime implies also a decrease of pauperism and taxation. An effective check upon rowdyism and vice on Sundays makes its influence felt through the whole week, saves to the labouring man his hard earnings, and adds to the comfort and happiness of his family.

"Many have already been converted to the Excise Law by these practical arguments. A German working-man, who used to spend his Sundays in the beer saloons, on being asked recently, on a Monday, how he felt, replied: 'Very well; I have no headache to-day, and no black eyes. I have my pocket full of money, and can comfortably support my family during the week.' A large German manufacturer says, that since the enforcement of the Excise Law, his employés come to the shop early on Monday morning, in good health and spirits, while before they came late, half drunk and unfit for work. At first, they abused the law, but now they feel the benefit and are contented with it.

All the churches are gainers by such a state of things. The superintendent of the New York City Mission and Tract Society states that 'this law is sending men by the score to our mission stations who never came before.'"*

Legislation so beneficial in its results cannot fail to commend itself to every unprejudiced person. It is strange how any one, with the facts before him and with the opportunity of observation, can oppose legislation requiring the orderly and decent observance of the Sabbath.

But it is said all men do not observe the same day as the Sabbath. The Jews and a few professing Christians observe Saturday. Mohammedans keep Friday. Hence, if the state enjoin the observance of any particular day, it does not respect the rights of conscience; and if it visit with penalty the infraction of its ordinance, it violates these rights.

The objection, if admitted, would lead to this absurd conclusion, that the state must not legislate with reference to any moral or religious institution concerning the moral and religious character of which men differ in opinion. Some consider polygamy to be right: must the state, then, decline to legislate concerning marriage? The Thugs of India believe murder to be right: should any of

* The Tenth Year of the New York Sabbath Committee, with a sketch of its History from 1857 to 1867, pp. 22, 23. Document No. XXXIV.

them emigrate to our shores, ought our government, out of respect to their opinion, to repeal the law against murder? The Hindoo mother considers it a religious act to cast her child into the Ganges: should a Christian government frame laws in accordance with her perverted religious sentiment, and suffer infanticide to go unpunished?

We are a Christian nation, and our legislation should be in harmony with the principles of Christianity. These principles, so far as they relate directly to legislation, are contained in the Decalogue, every law of which is of binding authority and cannot be set aside.

But does not the Fourth Commandment of the Decalogue enjoin the observance of the seventh day as a Sabbath—the very day observed as such by the Jews and some Christians? It does. But nearly all Christendom believes, for sufficient reasons, that the Sabbath, after the resurrection of Christ, was changed from the seventh day of the week to the first; and that this change is to continue until the end of the world. Those who keep the seventh day do not violate any positive command, but they do not conform to the example of the Apostles and of the primitive church. That example nearly all Christians consider binding: hence they feel it to be a duty to abstain from all secular employments on the first day of the week, and to spend it as a day of holy rest. Consequently they are excluded from all public works and service that require a violation of the Christian Sabbath, and denied an equality of rights with Jews and infidels. Should such a thing exist in a Christian land?

But it may be asked, would not the Jew be denied equality of rights by legislation protecting the Christian Sabbath and ignoring the Jewish? The answer is: We are not a Jewish, but a Christian nation; therefore, our legislation must be conformed to the institutions and spirit of Christianity. This is absolutely necessary from the nature of the case. A Christian nation cannot, without the greatest wrong to itself, ignore Christianity, or place it on a level with Judaism, Mohammedanism, and infidelity. Christianity is the salt of the earth —the great conservative principle of all that is good and holy in the world; and the Sabbath is the great conservator of Christianity.

Let us, then, preserve the Sabbath. Our highest interests require it. Our duty to ourselves as a Christian people, and to the many foreigners, who seek a home among us, demands it. Unless we are faithful in maintaining the institutions of Christianity our glory will depart; "for the nation and kingdom that will not serve thee shall perish; yea, those nations shall be utterly wasted." Is. lx. 12.

"What true heart loves not the Sabbath?
That dear pledge of home;
That trysting-place of God and man;
That link between a near eternity and time;
That almost lonely rivulet, which flows
From Eden through the world's wide wastes of sand

Unchecked, and, though not unalloyed with earth,
Its healing waters all impregned with life,
The life of their first blessing, to pure lips
The memory of a by-gone paradise,
The earnest of a paradise to come."

SECTION VI.

CONCLUDING REMARKS.

The subject of Sabbath sanctification is one of great practical importance, and affords of itself a theme for an extended treatise. The discussion of it in this little volume is necessarily limited: its main objects and points have only been indicated. The general heads, under which the special duties may be ranged, have been given. The devout mind, with the Bible for his guide and the Holy Spirit for his teacher, can determine for himself the details of duty appropriate to himself in his peculiar circumstances. The obligation of moral law is universal and permanent, but the mode of discharging that obligation is often affected by the condition and relations of the individual. Hence the application of general principles to specific cases would lead to much tedious detail. For this reason the author has confined himself to the discussion of general topics, which, however meagre the discussion may be, are sufficiently comprehensive.

www.ingramcontent.com/pod-product-compliance
Lightning Source LLC
LaVergne TN
LVHW021429110826
845150LV00007B/2159

* 9 7 8 1 4 2 5 5 0 7 2 8 2 *